Praise for
Eat, Live, Thrive Diet

"This book contains cutting-edge information to revolutionize your health and well-being! Health and weight loss is best done by addressing the total woman—body, soul, and spirit. *Eat, Live, Thrive Diet* gives accurate and practical insights and applications that will help women not only lose unwanted weight but also enhance their health in ways that could produce anti-aging results."
　　　—DR. MARK STENGLER, naturopathic medical doctor, best-selling author, and adviser
　　　　to *Eat, Live, Thrive Diet*

"This is not a book of theory; it's a practical, day-by-day manual on living your best life. If, like me, you want to have a strong, healthy body to serve God for as long as you can, this book is a gift."
　　　—SHEILA WALSH, author of *It's Okay Not to Be Okay*

"In *Eat, Live, Thrive Diet,* Danna and Robyn have passionately researched, lived, and committed themselves to sharing trailblazing information to inspire women to soar over the increasing physical hurdles they experience as they age. They give us hope that we can *thrive* beautifully as we dance with the years."
　　　—PATTI T. MILLIGAN, PhD, RD, CNS, natural foods and integrative medicine nutritionist

"Danna and Robyn have provided a road map for a sustainable lifestyle. Proof that our best bodies—and lives—are still ahead of us, no matter our age."
　　　—NANCY STAFFORD, actress, speaker, and author

"In this timely book, Danna and Robyn bring clarity to the guesswork, confusion, and contradictions that have puzzled eternal dieters over the years. Their candor, practicality, and encouragement bring renewed hope for all who want to glorify God with their bodies. This is a classic must-read!"
　　　—DEBORAH SMITH PEGUES, CPA, TV host, global speaker, and best-selling author

"Danna and Robyn have created a practical, encouraging, and vital resource that every woman needs to take her health and vitality to the next level. If you want to live longer and stronger, and be more vibrant, you should read this transforming book!"
　　　—PAM FARREL, codirector of Love-Wise and best-selling author

"I am now down more than thirty-seven pounds since the first of the year and have set my second goal to lose thirty-five more on this plan, and I feel so much better! I just returned Saturday from a week's vacation and am happy to say I did not gain a pound, thanks to tips from these two! In fact, when I weighed myself Monday morning, I was down a pound more!"

—LaCretia, a participant of the Eat, Live, Thrive Diet and Lifestyle Plan

"I was fifty-six years old and twenty-five pounds overweight. I was tired of carrying around menopausal weight that would not budge, no matter how hard I tried or what diet I chose. Then I stumbled onto this diet plan. After the first week, the weight began to budge and I felt better. My hair began to grow thicker and wasn't dry anymore, and my skin had a healthy shine. At about thirty days into this diet, I decided to develop an intermittent fasting routine that fit easily with my lifestyle. Then the weight and inches started coming off even more easily. I had increased energy and felt healthy again, something I had not experienced for more than ten years. Within six months, I lost twenty-five pounds and twenty-eight overall inches. Now, one year later, I've easily kept all the weight and inches off. I feel as if I've rolled the clock back twenty years."

—Sandi Thys, a participant of the Eat, Live, Thrive Diet and Lifestyle Plan

"I have known Danna for the past twenty years. She has a unique ability to speak to the need of body, soul, and spirit, giving her a strong practical impact. *Eat, Live, Thrive Diet* will help the individual looking for a significant change in their life to move forward. No fad approach here, just helpful tools to change the course of your life."

—Dr. Tim Scott, president of Hope Rescue, Inc.

"Danna and Robyn were instrumental in advising me in the rebuilding of my wellness after a bout of foodborne illness. They helped me discover things my doctors could not, and my gut is thankful! I could not wait to read this book. They confirmed hunches I have had for years about the connection between my brain and my stomach. The research is thorough and fascinating. And their hearts are beautiful. This book feels like a personal coaching experience with the world's foremost experts in body wellness for women, but it also feels like a fun conversation with two girlfriends!"

—Dannah Gresh, best-selling author of *Lies Girls Believe: And the Truth That Sets Them Free* and founder of True Girl

EATLIVETHRIVE DIET

A LIFESTYLE PLAN to REV UP YOUR MIDLIFE METABOLISM

DANNA DEMETRE AND ROBYN THOMSON

WATERBROOK

Library of Congress Cataloging-in-Publication Data
Names: Demetre, Danna, author. | Thomson, Robyn, author.
Title: Eat, live, thrive diet : a lifestyle plan to rev up your midlife metabolism / by Danna Demetre and Robyn Thomson.
Description: First Edition. | Colorado Springs: WaterBrook, 2019. | Includes bibliographical references.
Identifiers: LCCN 2018035604| ISBN 9780525653165 (pbk.) | ISBN 9780525653172 (electronic)
Subjects: LCSH: Weight loss. | Reducing diets—Recipes. | Health behavior. | Food habits—Psychological aspects. | Lifestyles—Health aspects. | Middle-aged women—Health and hygiene.
Classification: LCC RM222.2 .D459 2019 | DDC 613.2/5—dc23
LC record available at https://lccn.loc.gov/2018035604

Printed in the United States of America
2019—First Edition

10 9 8 7 6 5 4 3 2 1

This book is dedicated to every woman who has believed the lie that her best body, health, and life are in the past. We're here to shout from the rooftops that your best years can be ahead of you when you put the Eat, Live, Thrive Diet and Lifestyle Plan into action!

Contents

Introduction

We have a friend named Sarah. She recently had an epiphany, and she doesn't like it. "Oh my gosh. I've got a muffin top. I have no energy, and my body feels ten years older than I really am." Sarah sighed. "I've become my mother!"

Have you ever felt like that? As though your best years are behind you and you'll never feel even close to how vibrant you did in years past?

Well, we're here to tell you, "Stop thinking that way!"

It's true that for many women weight gain and lack of energy make them feel old. Their skin lacks the youthful glow and smoothness it once had. And if that weren't enough, dealing with perimenopause and postmenopause is not a cakewalk either.

Are you like Sarah, forty-five or older, with numerous diets under your belt, so to speak? And you still can't shed that extra layer of fat around your waist or thighs? We admit that it does get harder to lose weight and keep it off as we age. But it is not impossible!

We know because we've personally been in the trenches as you have. Maybe we haven't experienced exactly the same things, but we do understand "the struggle"!

Danna's Story

I still remember the despair I felt years ago that expressed itself in a nightmare. In my dream, I was shoving cookies, doughnuts, potato chips, and candy into my mouth at an alarming speed. I could not stop eating everything in sight. In the middle of my dream, I sat up in bed and yelled, "You. Just. Eat when you're hungry!" And then I flopped back down onto my pillow and started crying.

It didn't take a psychologist to unravel my inner turmoil. I dreamed this because it was my reality. By the time I was twenty years old, I'd been secretly binge eating for more than three years. Some days I ate enough to feed a small country. The reason I was only twenty-five pounds overweight rather than a hundred was because I purged.

By the time I was in my junior year of nursing school, I sometimes binged and purged five times a day. I was a physical and emotional wreck and had no idea how to get well. To top it off, I started to take amphetamines to try to control my urges, but they made me nervous and I couldn't sleep. I cycled for a long time between starvation on pills and bingeing.

No one knew I was bulimic. No one knew my pain. Not even my fiancé. I thought I was alone in my problem. Back in the 1970s, people talked about anorexia but not much about bulimia. I felt as though I was the biggest loser on the planet, and I wanted to die.

Then the panic attacks started.

Initially, they came only occasionally, but soon they were triggered by any stress—even leaving the house. I became a hypochondriac, always thinking the worst. My stomachache was an ulcer; my heart palpitations, a heart defect; my nervousness, low blood sugar. The list went on and on. Over time, I became convinced I was either dying or losing my mind.

I got A's in all my medical-surgical classes in nursing school as I attempted to diagnose myself. Then I shifted my attention to my mental health and got A's in psychology as I became convinced that I was suffering from one or more disorders. Medical doctors, counselors, psychologists—I saw them all. The panic attacks continued so intensely that I lived on high doses of Valium to calm me down enough to get through my classes and complete college.

In retrospect, living in fear and shame for all those years was the worst and best thing that ever happened to me. I know that sounds weird, but let me explain.

As my panic attacks went from uncomfortable, free-floating anxiety to terrorizing moments when I seriously believed I was dying, I was forced to ask myself, *What would happen if I did die?*

I was utterly exhausted from living in constant fear. One night, I was home alone and had the most severe panic attack I'd ever experienced. I was certain something was terribly wrong with me and I was going to die all alone in my bedroom.

Having been a nurse, I realize I was probably hyperventilating so much that I was in danger of passing out—but certainly not of dying. I remember sitting on the edge of my bed and burying my face in my hands, trying to breathe slowly and calm myself. I cried out to a God I believed in but did not truly know. I believed he existed, but I had no idea how to reach him or if he heard my feeble cries.

Well, he did. In that moment he brought a woman to my mind—the one and only woman in my life I would have called "religious." I found her phone number in my address book and called her that very moment. In a breathless rant, I told her that I was dying and needed to know if she knew God personally. You have to be rather desperate to do that. I was.

Sweet Tonette assured me that she not only knew God but that God knew *me*. This godly, selfless woman poured into me over the next days and weeks and shared the gospel with me. I found a new, saving faith in Jesus Christ. While he did not heal me instantly of my fear, bulimia, and insecurities, he did begin a healing process in me and I learned the power of a renewed mind. (I'll share more about that in chapter 3.)

Today in my midsixties, I am leaner than I was in my thirties. I'm often told I look fifteen to twenty years younger than I am. I don't know about that, but I do know that I *feel* that young and that life is so much richer as my health and vitality continue to soar.

Regardless of what kind of battle you're in, there is hope for victory. Perhaps you've simply developed some unhealthy habits that need to be exchanged for healthier ones. Or maybe you feel as though you've lost all control when it comes to food. No matter. Change is possible!

Robyn's Story

I was chubby as a child and adolescent. I remember being teased about my size and feeling self-conscious and inadequate compared to the other girls at my school. Then one summer in my early teens, I experienced a massive growth spurt and shed all my excess body fat, just like that.

My classmates didn't even recognize me when I returned to school in the fall. Their acceptance of me based on my outward appearance was quite eye opening. I knew that I never wanted to be overweight again.

I stayed lean and was very content with my body into my twenties and thirties. But when I hit my forties, something changed. I started gaining weight, even though I was doing the same things I'd always done.

I realized quickly that I couldn't eat the same way I had and was determined not to travel full circle and become a chubby menopausal woman. I knew I would need to make some strategic changes quickly, but I had no idea what those changes should be.

To add insult to injury, the quest to drop the excess pounds was even more challenging because I began to experience an unexplainable and insatiable hunger. I would finish a full and normally satisfying meal and then would want to eat a second one before I left the table! Thankfully, I did not give in to my feelings, but the sensation of always being hungry became stronger and more disturbing. And to make it even more unfair, eating made me even hungrier!

I have seen many doctors over the years, including my primary-care physician, two endocrinologists, and my naturopathic medical doctor, who is brilliant and very skilled at getting to the root of many hormonal and metabolic issues. He's truly perplexed that everything we try seems to fail.

All the pros do agree on one thing: this is not an emotional issue but rather a physiological one, particularly that hormonal signals between my stomach and my brain may not be getting through. Oh my!

Though I've found many creative ways to manage this "thorn in the flesh," so far there's no complete and lasting solution. It is still something I face every single day, some days more intensely than others.

My challenge with weight gain and relentless hunger sparked a focused motivation to find answers. I've committed the past decade to massive research to find the best diet and supplements to become and stay lean as a woman over fifty.

I've also learned the importance of trusting God in the journey. He gives me the strength not to cave in to the lies my body tells me about being hungry. By his grace, and a strong foundation of personal discipline, I've stayed my ideal size through most of my "hunger games." On the rare occasions when my weight has crept up, I've taken drastic action, such as fasting for thirty-six hours to break the cycle.

I must choose my goal over immediate gratification hour by hour. It's a skill I've developed over time, and I've surprised myself by how strong I can be with God's help. He does his part, but I must also do mine! The alternative—giving in to my hunger—would result in obesity.

I use many of the nonfood techniques we teach in our Eat, Live, Thrive Diet as tools to help me choose well. If I can do it—with relentless hunger—you can do it too.

I know and believe this completely. It is our job to help you believe it as well!

I won't pretend that my hunger issue hasn't been hard. Do I get discouraged? Sure I do! Do I get frustrated? Daily. Sometimes I'm so weary trying to find a solution that I wonder, *Why can't I just be satisfied?* On occasion I succumb to my strong desire to eat, even though I know that my body does not need more food. Usually I eat foods that are healthy, but other times, not so much. I may be a nutrition expert and weight-loss coach, but I'm also human!

I share all this because I want you to know that you don't need to be a victim of your "feelings." Danna and I had very different challenges. Hers was mental and emotional; mine was physical. We both needed to make an important decision about how we would respond to our respective challenges. Would we give up, or would we be proactive?

We chose action, and you can too!

Everyone Has a Story

You have a story too, and it is important. It gives you perspective and motivates you to give yourself grace for being human. But your history (the past) does not need to be an excuse for staying stuck (in the present)! We are certain that you can rewrite your story in a way that brings you a sense of victory and freedom, and we want to help you do that.

After reading our stories, you can tell we both have a strong faith in God. Perhaps you share our Christian faith; perhaps you don't. Although we do share teaching that applies to not only the body and mind but the spiritual dimension as well, most of the principles mentioned are universal truths that can be applied and produce great results regardless of religious belief.

This Book Is for You!

We're honored that you've chosen to go on this journey with us to discover how to eat, live, and thrive no matter your age. The Eat, Live, Thrive Diet and Lifestyle Plan is for all women, with extra help for women over forty-five because of the unique challenges that emerge as we age.

We wish we'd known some of these strategies much earlier in our lives. Practicing them will help you stay "ageless" into midlife and beyond. We like the word *ageless* over *mature* because it reflects both an attitude and a lifestyle that defy time. We're excited for you to take this journey with us so you can celebrate life fully in the years ahead.

In part 1, we want to prepare you for long-term success by addressing various challenges and strategies before we dig into the three phases of the Eat, Live, Thrive Diet. However, if you are chomping at the bit and want to start Phase 1 of the diet today, you certainly have "permission" to skip ahead to part 2. Today is always the best time to take action! However, make sure you return to part 1 once you're underway because one of the most important chapters in the book—"You Are What You Think" (chapter 3)—provides simple steps for permanently overcoming some of the challenges you've probably faced over the years when trying to lose weight and keep it off. Plus, the concept of short-term fasting and the reasons why we've designed an eating cycle specifically for ageless women is also clarified in part 1. You may also want to visit our support website and watch our "Getting Started" video at EatLiveThriveDiet.com.

Whatever you believe, whatever you've experienced, wherever you are in your life journey, we want you to know that you can benefit from the Eat, Live, Thrive (ELT) strategy and tips we share to help you rev up your midlife metabolism, lighten the scale, and turn back the clock.

Now let's get introduced to the Eat, Live, Thrive Diet and Lifestyle Plan!

PART 1

PREPARATION

Eat: To nourish your body and embrace your God-given sense of taste.

Live: To fully experience the abundant life.

Thrive: To flourish in body, soul, and spirit.

We are all so different. If Danna burns more calories than she eats, she sheds fat and her weight goes down. Not so for Robyn. Like many (perhaps most) women over forty-five, she is highly sensitive to grains. But unlike many women, Robyn is not insulin resistant, so she can eat a normal amount of carbohydrates and still lose weight. She just can't include many grains or legumes because her body hates them and revolts by triggering digestive symptoms, water retention, mental fogginess, and weight gain.

In contrast to both of us, our friend Janice can barely look at a starchy carbohydrate without gaining weight. She is highly insulin resistant. More on that to come, but it means that her muscle cells don't allow insulin to transport carbohydrates (converted into glucose) to be stored (as glycogen) for future energy. Because survival requires that glucose not accumulate in the blood, it gets diverted to Janice's fat cells, which happily convert it to more fat. Even when she eats what she considers normal amounts of grains and other starches, such as potatoes, Janice gains weight.

Counting calories does not work for Janice. Fortunately, the Eat, Live, Thrive Diet does.

Like the three of us, you are unique. So what are *your* dietary

> God has provided us with a sophisticated healing system. Focus on the building blocks of what he has provided, such as sound nutrition, exercise, sleep, attitude, and prayer.
>
> —Mark Stengler, NMD

stumbling blocks? These can be difficult to figure out on your own. The ELT Diet can help you discover the foods that are holding you back from reaching your goals.

The Reality of Weight Gain After Forty-Five

Women over forty-five are often faced with these issues when it comes to weight loss:
- a lower carbohydrate threshold, which declines steadily with age
- insulin resistance, which increases over time and promotes diabetes
- unknown food sensitivities
- hormonal imbalance
- slower metabolism due to muscle atrophy

After the age of thirty, we lose the ability to utilize and burn carbohydrates as well as we did when we were younger. The decline is slow and insidious and can go unnoticed into our forties and perhaps fifties, but it is happening. Foods that we once could eat are now causing undue inflammation in our bodies and are disrupting our digestion, joint health, and metabolism.

All the while, as we are edging toward menopause—or in the midst of it or past it—our hormones are being greatly influenced by many of the grains and processed foods we eat, making it more difficult to maintain any level of hormone balance even if we are using the latest and greatest bioidentical hormones and supplements.

That's the reality. What can we do about it?

The ABCs of the ELT Diet

If you want to be lean and healthy, look younger than your birth certificate indicates, and have the energy to embrace life fully, you must nourish your body with real food. Our diet plan will help you not only burn fat and drop pounds but also rev up your energy. It also provides a nutritional foundation to slow down and perhaps even reverse some of the aging process.

Our ELT Diet and Lifestyle Plan is designed to

Activate your metabolism and promote steady weight loss

Balance your blood sugar and cravings

Cleanse your body of toxins and decrease inflammation

Our eating plan is especially effective for mature (ageless!) women who've experienced continued difficulty losing weight on portion- or calorie-controlled diets. It is strategically designed to promote a robust metabolism, which enhances fat-burning capability no matter one's age. Our participants are amazed at how much they can eat on our diet and still get excellent and steady results.

Step-by-Step Guidance

In the ELT Diet and Lifestyle Plan, we will guide you through three progressive phases, culminating in a realistic *and* enjoyable lifestyle eating plan that will serve you well for the rest of your life.

We'll show you how to use the first two phases to reboot your lifestyle when you veer a bit off track. (Let's be honest—who doesn't? Our strategies help you address that reality so you can keep moving forward.)

We will teach you how to make your body shift from being predominantly a carbohydrate or sugar burner to a metabolically agile burner of all fuels, including fat.

We'll introduce you to the power of intermittent fasting and all its benefits and our kinder and gentler version called the Eat, Live, Thrive Eating Cycle. While short-term fasting is optional, we know from our own personal experiences and from the testimonies of many of our clients that it can be a game changer. And the benefits go far beyond weight loss. The benefits extend to brain health, higher energy, and disease prevention.

And just as important, we'll teach you how to design a lasting lifestyle eating plan that will be your foundation for life. Yes, there's room for a few empty calories. No, you won't follow your ideal plan perfectly every day. But you will discover the best plan for you and know that if you practice it moderately well most days, your body will reward you with great results!

Although our diet was designed specifically for women, it works great for men as well. We've been pleased to learn that many husbands and boyfriends are so impressed with their wives' and girlfriends' weight loss and health improvement that they decide to try the diet too. They love the recipes and healthy substitutions we recommend to replace the foods that are troublesome. But beware: men lose weight faster than women, so don't let that discourage you!

Figuring Out Good and Bad Foods

After years of coaching women, we have seen the greatest breakthroughs when specific troublesome foods are eliminated for a period of time and then reintroduced strategically based on the body's response. Most women have no idea that they have a sensitivity to certain foods because they've not identified a direct correlation between the food and its negative effect on their bodies.

It has been documented that more than 20 percent of people in industrialized countries have food intolerances that disrupt their health and contribute to weight-loss challenges.[1] Additionally, it is estimated that approximately 65 percent of adults have some level of lactose intolerance.[2] It is impossible to know how many undocumented sensitivities exist considering the steadily increasing number of individuals struggling with leaky gut and other digestive issues. And quite frankly, most of us are simply consuming too many processed foods and realizing the effects of all the additives and preservatives.

Some women don't remember what it's like to feel great. They have no clue that removing certain foods and adding others can help them look and feel years younger. Just imagine turning back your biological clock by simply eating the right foods for you. It is not only possible but also relatively easy to discover how to do just that using the personalized approach we teach in this book.

An Almost-New Body Every Eight Years

God designed our bodies with perfect blueprints that tell them what to do with the fuel we give them. They know how to build new blood cells, skin, muscles, bones, and so on. In fact, our bodies are constantly regenerating. We slough off dead skin cells hourly and replace them with new ones. We regenerate red blood cells within 120 days. We even build an entirely new skeletal system over time.

Unbelievably, the majority of living cells in your body today will not be present in your body eight years from now![3]

Just as you cannot build a brick house out of straw, you cannot build a healthy body out of chocolate chip cookies and potato chips. The quality of the skin, bones, muscles, and cells of your body depends on the quality of the building materials you choose to supply, meal after meal! You truly are (and will be) what you eat.

We hope that this fact will motivate you to see each food you put in your body for what it is and that you'll choose wisely based on what you learn as you experience the ELT Diet.

Beyond Gluten Sensitivity

Many have jumped on the gluten-free bandwagon, and for good reason. It is estimated that much of the Western world is showing signs of being highly sensitive to an overabundance of processed wheat products. These include commercially made breads, pastas, crackers, packaged sauces, salad dressings, and, of course, desserts.

Many of the most well-respected health experts believe that there are no significant nutritional benefits found in commercially made wheat products and that everyone would be better served by removing them from their diets. Patti Milligan, the ELT Diet's functional nutrition adviser and a registered dietician with a master's degree in nutritional biochemistry and exercise science, agrees. She believes that the quality of mainstream wheat products in the US is troublesome for everyone—not just those with an actual sensitivity to wheat—because conventional wheat is washed in chlorine. Additionally, many packaged wheat products use additives and preservatives that wreak havoc on our bodies.

Unfortunately, the solution is not just to go gluten free. Many people make the shift to gluten free but then end up eating excessive amounts of corn- or rice-based products, which also creates a high carbohydrate load and other challenges for their bodies. Additionally, food sensitivities go far beyond gluten. Many of our clients are flabbergasted to realize that some of the "healthy" foods they've been eating are problems for them.

Even when true sensitivity is not an issue, sugar addiction, carbohydrate overload, and toxic buildup (from all the commercially processed foods) can send our bodies into a downward health spiral. Strategically eliminating food culprits and testing each to determine our reactions are key in discovering the ideal diet for our bodies.

> In the Western world, we eat the quantity of carbohydrates as if we're training for a marathon, but we never run the marathon!
>
> —Patti Milligan

Therefore, if you have cut calories and still not lost weight, reduced all fat and gotten fatter, exercised your tail off and the fat hasn't budged, watched the fat around your middle increase over the past decade, gained and lost and gained and lost, *then it's time to turn your attention to the type and quality of foods you eat regularly.* Also, it is very likely you're exceeding your carbohydrate threshold and converting those calories quickly to stored fat.

Insulin Resistance and Beyond

Excessive carbohydrate intake and insufficient carbohydrate metabolism (in other words, insulin resistance) are at the root of many women's weight issues. Patti Milligan believes the average woman consumes about 300 to 350 grams of total carbohydrates per day. That amounts to almost 1,400 calories in carbohydrates alone, which is about 82 percent of a woman's total caloric needs for one day.[4]

Insulin resistance (IR), also known as metabolic syndrome, can range from minimal to extreme. It is a progressive disease if not treated with proper diet modifications. It has become synonymous with prediabetes. IR puts you at high risk of developing type 2 diabetes, and it triples your risk for heart disease. Losing weight becomes almost impossible unless you change your diet consistently.

Your body must maintain a very narrow blood-sugar (glucose) range at all times. Blood-sugar spikes occur when you consume more carbohydrates than necessary to meet *immediate* energy requirements. When this happens, the excess glucose produced must be promptly transported and stored elsewhere. That is the job of insulin. It converts that excess into either glycogen (an energy source stored in the muscles or liver) or fat. Fat becomes the primary storage if glycogen stores are full and/or you are insulin resistant.

IR is caused when muscle, liver, and fat cells do not respond effectively to insulin. Research reveals that this problem increases as we age and is closely related to lifestyle habits. The most important of these habits is the quality of our nutrition. That means we can have control over this ever-increasing metabolic syndrome by changing our diets.

Approximately 50 percent of Americans have some form of insulin resistance, according to Dr. Robert Lustig, professor of pediatric endocrinology at the University of California, San Francisco.[5] That percentage is even higher in adults older than forty-five. "In contrast to popular false beliefs, weight loss and health should not be a constant battle uphill through calorie restriction, which simply doesn't work," says Dr. Andreas Eenfeldt in an article on his blog. He then goes on to quote Dr. Lustig:

> Following current dietary advice is counterintuitive to achieving a healthy weight.
>
> The reason is the myth of energy balance. If you believe this, then you believe that obesity is a physics problem; too much energy in, too little energy out. Energy balance assumes that all calories are equal, no matter where they come from. Rather, obesity is about energy

---

An individual is considered to have insulin resistance (IR) if he or she has three or more of the following markers:
- blood pressure ≥ 130/85 mm Hg or use of medication for hypertension
- fasting glucose ≥ 100 mg/dL or use of medication for high blood glucose
- HDL cholesterol ≤ 50 mg/dL
- triglycerides ≥ 150 mg/dL
- waist circumference ≥ 35 inches

---

deposition into fat tissue. Obesity is a biochemistry problem, and where those nutrients came from determine where they go in the body. It's called nutritional biochemistry and it shows that all calories are not created equal.[6]

Even for women who are not truly insulin resistant, excessive carbohydrates can create a roller-coaster effect as blood-sugar levels peak and then fall throughout the day. Thus, cravings increase, energy decreases, and immunity declines.

Patti Milligan also alerts us to the important role that a sedentary lifestyle plays in insulin resistance. Just increasing movement to three ten-minute spurts of intentional activity within your day can significantly improve your cells' sensitivity to insulin because it stokes your metabolic furnace. In chapter 12, we'll share the importance of leading an active lifestyle and tips to easily improve your fitness.

Now let's take a look at an overview of the three key phases of the ELT Diet and Lifestyle Plan.

Small steps taken *consistently* add up in a big way over time!

—Danna

Here's the bad news: about 30 percent of our health and vitality is out of our control because of our genetics and gender. You may have genetic predispositions to certain diseases or metabolic challenges. As a woman, you have various hormone shifts through the years that you cannot avoid.

But here's the good news: 70 percent is in your control!

That 70 percent is called your *lifestyle,* and it makes a much bigger impact on your future than you may think.

How you choose to eat, exercise, sleep, relax, and deal with stress adds up in big ways. Don't rely on "good genes" to get you by long term. You can have the best genes on the planet, but if you don't take good care of yourself, you will age more quickly than necessary and succumb to many diseases that are quite preventable.

Of all your lifestyle choices, what you eat will have the most bearing. You can exercise regularly and sleep like a teenager, but over the long haul, it is the food you eat that will most influence your health and well-being. As Dr. Josh Axe puts it so succinctly, "Food is medicine"![1]

In contrast, much of what we eat may be edible and give our bodies energy, but these foods do not nurture health and can cause our bodies significant "dis-ease."

Eat, Live, Thrive to the Rescue

We need to address this epidemic directly, and that's why we've created the Eat, Live, Thrive Diet and Lifestyle Plan. And we start with the *short-term* elimination of all processed foods, grains, and sugar. Doing this will immediately give your body a full respite from the stress and strain of your current diet.

The Eat, Live, Thrive Plan includes three phases:

1. The Elimination Phase
2. The Discovery Phase
3. The Lifestyle Phase

At the end of each diet-phase chapter, we include a synopsis with specific success steps you can take to keep each phase very simple. We also provide worksheets to help you reach your daily goals. Studies show that journaling or using some form of log promotes lasting weight-loss success. You can download these worksheets at EatLiveThriveDiet.com. Simply register with your email address to obtain unlimited access.

1. The Elimination Phase

The program begins with the temporary elimination of several key foods known to promote insulin resistance and cause allergies, sensitivities, and inflammation. By removing these foods from their diet for at least fourteen days, most women lose weight without calorie counting or portion control. They enjoy eating to satisfaction from the list of approved foods at each level.

This stage in the diet can be followed safely for longer than fourteen days—actually for as long as you like—and it is the phase in which you will notice the most weight loss. We'll discuss this more in chapter 7.

We understand that life can be busy and complicated. We also recognize that there are emotional and logistic challenges that may hamper your ability to participate at the highest level. Therefore, we've provided three different options for the Elimination Phase to suit your current needs. We'll describe them later. But one note: if you don't start at Level 3 (the highest), we recommend that you do move toward that level at some point so you experience the most dramatic benefits possible.

And don't worry—there's a place for some starches and treats in your long-term diet. How many? That's what we will discover together. It depends on your unique carbohydrate threshold, food sensitivities, activity level, stress load, and resting metabolic rate.

We'll help you breeze through this phase without a lot of cravings because the diet will help balance your blood sugar and our recipes are designed to keep you satisfied. You'll find them near the back of the book in part 5, starting on page 186. They've received rave reviews from our clients who continue to use them on a regular basis. And a bonus is that most family members love them as well.

Of course, you can also use your own recipes if all the ingredients are on the approved food list of the diet level you choose.

2. The Discovery Phase

The next phase, the Discovery Phase, is an adventure because it is an opportunity for you to discover why you experienced weight loss and health benefits during the Elimination Phase. The Discovery Phase is essential for your long-term success because you can lock in the results you achieved in Phase 1.

By reintroducing each eliminated food—one at a time—you will be able to determine which specific foods are troublesome for you. Some may cause immediate weight gain, inflammation, digestive upset, or other symptoms. Others may not produce any negative symptoms until you've had a few servings, so you may be able to eat these foods moderately on occasion.

You will also discover if eating more grains or carbohydrates in general causes you to quickly gain back the weight you lost. This can be the case if you have a lowered carbohydrate threshold or full-blown insulin resistance. The only way to know for sure is to eliminate, reintroduce, and carefully monitor your reaction. You'll learn more about this in chapter 8.

The Discovery Phase will very likely reveal some of the missing links to reaching your health and weight-loss goals. But if life gets in the way and you cannot complete the full Discovery Phase by testing all the potentially troublesome foods, test what you can for this first cycle. Then when life is more manageable, restart the process with a minimum seven days of elimination and test the remaining foods.

We recommend taking three days to test each food. If you have a negative reaction, you need to wait to test the next food until all symptoms are gone. The entire Discovery Phase can potentially take a month or more, depending on your reactions and the number of foods you've chosen to eliminate.

You may go through Phases 1 and 2 of the diet several times and discover something new each time. Remember: this is a journey of discovery that you can repeat and perfect as you gain new understanding about your body.

3. The Lifestyle Phase

Once you know which foods trip you up, you can begin to design an ideal long-term eating plan that accommodates your specific needs and preferences. In chapter 9, we make the process for the Lifestyle Phase super easy.

We've included thought-provoking questions to help you pinpoint your goals and greatest challenges. You'll have specific guidelines and two approaches to choose from: "Keep It Simple" or "By the Numbers."

Make the Program Work for You

One of our mottoes is Progress, Not Perfection. Change takes time. Following the diet phases "perfectly" may be ideal but is also unrealistic. When you can make several consistent changes most days, the occasional slipup will not set you back too much. Over time, it will get easier and easier to make healthier choices, and a leaner, more youthful, and more energetic body will be a great motivator.

Learning how to design your own modifications and find creative ways to use the diet phases to suit your lifestyle will benefit you long term. We'll give you lots of examples of how to do that in the Lifestyle Phase. But before we dig into the specifics of the diet and its three phases, we want to address a very important topic: habits. Knowing *what* to do is not enough. Knowing *how* to get yourself to follow through and do it is essential. Yet few diets address this issue. In the next two chapters, we'll do just that.

From simple attitude adjustments to a major "mind renewal" overhaul, we'll share scientific facts about your brain and psychology, biblical principles, and practical tips both of us have used for decades to adopt and sustain healthy lifestyles. These practices work for us, and they can work for you as well!

> I do not understand what I do. For what I want to
> do I do not do, but what I hate I do.
>
> —ROMANS 7:15

Do these words from the apostle Paul resonate with you? Do you wonder why it is so hard to make yourself do the things you know are good for you? You are not alone.

We all struggle with the "battle of the flesh," and many of us succumb easily when it comes to food or other forms of immediate gratification. It's like there is an urge that cries out, "I want it. I need it. I've got to have it. Now!"

Making healthier choices is definitely easier said than done. Mustering an extra dose of willpower or motivation is not enough. We need to get to the core of the issue, which quite often is rooted in unhealthy thinking and bad habits. Our underlying perspective is more powerful than most of us realize.

In fact, the power of our thoughts influences us in so many ways we cannot begin to fathom, even changing our body chemistry!

Mind over Milkshake

Alia Crum, a clinical psychologist and assistant professor at Stanford University, wanted to know if a nutritional label could physically alter what happens to a person eating that food. She'd spent her early years as a student studying the placebo effect (i.e., how a sugar pill can physically alter a body if the person taking the pill believes it will).

In 2011 Crum devised an interesting new experiment using food. First, she made a large batch of French vanilla milkshake and then divided it into two. One batch was labeled as a low-calorie drink called "Sensishake." The label reflected that the drink had no fat or added sugar and was only 140 calories. The other batch was called "Indulgence." Its label indicated that the shake contained a high amount of sugar and fat to account for the whopping 620 calories. The reality: both shakes were a moderate 300 calories.

> Our beliefs matter in virtually every domain, in everything we do. How much is a mystery, but I don't think we've given enough credit to the role of our beliefs in determining our physiology, our reality. We have this very simple metabolic science: calories in, calories out. People don't want to think that our beliefs have influence, too. But they do!
>
> —Alia Crum, clinical psychologist

The people in the study had their ghrelin levels measured before and after they drank their version of the shake. Ghrelin is what many health pros call the hunger hormone. When levels of ghrelin rise in the stomach, this tells your brain that you are hungry and that it's time to find food. Metabolism also slows down in case the need for food is not met right away.

After a substantial meal, ghrelin levels will drop, signaling to your brain that you've had enough to eat, and your metabolism increases, allowing you to burn the new calories from the meal. If a meal or snack is small, the levels don't drop very much and the metabolism remains less robust.

Most scientists have assumed that ghrelin levels fluctuate in direct relation to the actual nutrients the ghrelin encounters in the stomach. That is not what Crum discovered in her milkshake study. This is what she reported:

The ghrelin levels dropped about three times more when people were consuming the indulgent shake (or thought they were consuming the indulgent shake), compared to the people who drank the sensible shake (or thought that's what they were drinking).[1]

Wow! The ghrelin levels dropped more just because the participants *thought* they were consuming an indulgent shake. Just imagine what could happen if you rewired your thinking to consider healthy choices as "indulgent"!

This eye-opening illustration should motivate us all to cultivate healthy mental habits for a lifetime.

The Freeways of the Mind

Our brains were designed by our Creator to respond in specific ways. And the brain—just like the heart, liver, and kidneys—is designed to perform certain vital functions. It's helpful to understand how God made this magnificent glob of gray matter work the way it does. We can better appreciate the complexity of our feelings and our behaviors when we understand the brain's physiology.

With recent advances in medical technology, researchers have come to better understand that the human brain has an almost unlimited capacity to store information. Before we are born, we begin to develop billions of neural pathways. These are complex, microscopic circuits where our thoughts and experiences create an explosion of electrical activity. And it is where all our mental data is stored.

Some of these pathways can become physically strong and dominant because the thought or experience is frequently repeated. They become like superhighways in our minds, overriding many of the weaker pathways or less dominant thoughts.

The size of our neural pathways can physically change. Old dominant pathways can shrink and become less influential when they are neglected or overridden with new messages. And smaller, weaker pathways can physically grow and become like superhighways. How? They change through repetition. You've heard the saying that practice makes perfect. More accurately, the statement should be that practice makes permanent. How perfect will depend on the quality of what is being practiced.

Stewardship of Our Minds

Like computers, our brains do not place judgment on their data. They just store information, true or false, day after day, week after week, month after month, year after year. Ultimately, we come to believe the strongest messages—those messages that have played the loudest and most frequently throughout our lives. But what if that information is wrong? Well, just imagine what would happen if someone replaced the data that is stored in the NASA computers with wrong information. The result would be disastrous. The same is true with our minds.

This is what author Bob George refers to in his book *Classic Christianity:* "People . . . are locked in error, and that error has them in emotional and physical bondage."[2]

From Bible scholars to the most popular modern-day motivational speakers, those who have studied human behavior know that *how we think* drives our choices and behavior. Though our brains function as storage centers for information, God has also given us the ability to think, reason, and apply knowledge.

God has, in effect, given us stewardship of our minds.

From our simplest habits to our most destructive behaviors, our actions are the direct results of our mental programming. Both psychologists and biblical scholars agree that it is almost impossible for individuals to behave inconsistently with what they believe about themselves. Your mind will naturally go in the direction of your most prevalent thoughts.

If this is true—and it is—there is no permanent way to change our behavior without first changing our minds. That's why diets alone tend to fail. All the change is external. And when the diet is over, 95 percent of people revert to old programmed behaviors.

It's essential to change the program!

If you don't like who you are, don't just change your behavior—change your thoughts. It may feel awkward at first, as though you're lying to yourself, but your brain doesn't know the difference. At a point, it will respond to that dominant message as if it were true.

Listen to yourself when you look in the mirror each morning. What words do you use as you resolve to lose that excess weight? How do you describe your body, your fitness, your energy, your self-control? If you keep telling yourself that you are fat and you hate exercise, you'll continue to believe it. Those beliefs will sabotage your efforts.

Most of us have heard that it takes 21 days to change a habit. Unfortunately, many experts now believe that it takes 21 days for any change to *begin* to take place. For most people, it takes much longer than that for a new habit to become fully established. A 2018 study evaluated ninety-six individuals and concluded that on average it takes 66 days for a new habit to become second nature. However, the individual timelines varied from 18 to 254 days.[3]

Renew Your Mind to Transform Your Body

Getting beneath the surface and discovering scriptural truths about who we are and how God sees us can help us overcome many of the lies we've been telling ourselves. Sometimes we know these truths intellectually but still don't believe them for ourselves.

As a new believer still struggling with panic attacks and bulimia, I (Danna) was excited the first time I read Romans 12:2, which says, "Do not conform to the pattern of this world, but be transformed by the renewing of your mind."

Wow, that sounded so good! *Transformed.* It's a powerful word. But how do we do it? In my journey toward wholeness, I learned that we are transformed by truth. When we see, hear, speak, and believe that truth over and over, it replaces the lies we've been believing.

In the first part of that verse, we are told not to conform to this world. What does that mean? Conforming means complying with a set of customs or standards. God calls us to be different and set apart rather than driven by our culture's values. This can be very hard to do, especially when we are bombarded with ideas and images that tell us how to think and be.

How God Renewed Danna's Mind

As I (Danna) shared in the introduction, my severe panic attacks and bulimia motivated me to begin a relentless journey to find truth. During those years of internal struggle, I doubted I would ever be free of the paralyzing fear and lack of control that permeated my life daily.

Do not underestimate what God may be doing in your own struggles to draw you closer to him and transform you into the woman he wants you to become. This battle of the body is so much more than a physical one, and God can use every aspect of your journey to his glory and your benefit.

In the first few weeks as a new believer, I was ravenous for answers to overcome my fear. I could hardly set down my Bible. One day while reading, I ran across a verse that made me catch my breath. It was like water in the desert to my thirsty soul. I felt as if it were written just for me. The verse is

---

Winning Thoughts

In the human brain, the most dominant thoughts win. So what are your dominant thoughts? Are they serving you well? Or have your persistent negative thoughts made you their unknowing servant?

Don't underestimate the power of truth to transform you from the inside out. As a starting point, copy these statements of affirmation and put them in a place where you will be reminded to review them every day:

- *I am excited to discover a healthier lifestyle and watch my body transform.*
- *I love being active, so I make exercise a part of my daily lifestyle.*
- *I choose to eat for maximum energy and health.*
- *I am changing my unhealthy beliefs and attitudes.*
- *I am becoming transformed by the renewing of my mind.*
- *I can see myself leaner and healthier in the months ahead.*

---

2 Timothy 1:7, and it says, "God has not given us a spirit of fear, but of power and of love and of a sound mind" (NKJV).

Every time I sensed a panic attack brewing, I would say this verse. I personalized it and said, "God has not given *me* a spirit of fear, but of power and of love and of a sound mind." I must have repeated those words thirty or forty times *each day* for six months.

At the same time, I began reminding myself of other truths. When I felt anxious, I would tell myself that God was with me and had never let me die or "fall off the edge" before. And even if I did die, at least I knew where I was going! Over the course of the next nine months, my panic episodes became less intense and less frequent. Before the end of a year, they were completely gone. Oh, the power of truth to transform us through the renewing of our minds!

Two things happened in my journey toward transformation. The first was physical. As I repeatedly counteracted the lies I believed about losing my mind, dying, and being out of control with the scripture and statements I've mentioned, my neural pathways started to change. My old, destructive, dominant pathways started to shrink, and the new messages created strong new pathways, which grew until they finally propelled me to have healthier feelings and behavior. And although the change was gradual, much like watching our hair grow, it was very real.

I believe the second thing that happened was supernatural. In Hebrews 4:12, it is explained like this: "The word of God is alive and active. Sharper than any double-edged sword, it penetrates even to dividing soul and spirit, joints and marrow; it judges the thoughts and attitudes of the heart."

Spiritual and Physical Transformation

God's Word, the Bible, is so much more than wisdom and good advice. It is alive! It is active and does surgery on our hearts and minds. The Greek word for "sword" in Hebrews is *machaira.* Biblical scholar Tim Scott, my pastor, told me that it means "a short dagger, like a double-edged surgical knife." As I pondered this text, I realized that I had turned the truth of God's Word on myself and allowed it to cut out the lies I believed and replace them with life-changing truth. When I exposed myself to and dwelled upon God's truth, it miraculously transformed me.

As with the changing of my neural pathways, there was no crash course or shortcuts. I just applied God's Word consistently to my life day after day, and in his perfect timing, I was transformed.

We promise that you can be transformed too.

The Power of Self-Talk

Change Your Thoughts, Change Your Habits

4

> The brain simply believes what you tell it most. And what you tell it about you, it will create. It has no choice.
>
> —SHAD HELMSTETTER

One of the most practical ways to begin the process of changing your thinking is to get in tune with your self-talk. That may sound a little New Age, but it's not. The truth is, we all talk to ourselves in the privacy of our own minds. Unfortunately, most of us aren't paying attention to what we are saying.

Have you ever had thoughts like these?

- *I'm so fat and ugly.*
- *I know God loves me.*
- *I hate myself!*
- *I've decided to change my lifestyle.*
- *I'm out of control.*
- *I'm in control of my choices.*
- *I deserve this chocolate.*
- *I think I can do it.*
- *I'm so stressed.*
- *I handle life stresses well and lean in to God.*
- *Why am I so depressed?*
- *I won't give up.*
- *I can't do it.*
- *I believe God will help me.*
- *I'm such a failure.*

Such statements reflect a mix of both positive and negative thoughts and feelings. Most of us are oblivious to the power these messages have in our lives. When we become intentional about guarding our minds and taking our thoughts captive, we can make tremendous positive steps toward dynamic and lasting change.

In his book *The Healing Power of a Christian Mind,* Dr. William Backus comments on this subject of self-talk:

> As a clinical psychologist and pastor, I've been well aware for decades how dark depressive thoughts and negative self-talk creates more emotional problems than the actual events that trigger our emotions. *Self-talk* refers to the way we mentally process events—that is, how we interpret things that happen to us. . . .
>
> That's why it's important to understand how our self-talk—those statements we make to ourselves—form our emotions: powerful feelings like fear, anger, worry. . . .
>
> Today, I am convinced that strengthening your spirit with the bold, encouraging, life-giving truths that are revealed in the Bible—God's Word—will help you move toward physical wholeness and overall well-being. . . .
>
> Your spirit communicates with your mind, and your mind communicates with your body. . . .
>
> The truth has a positive impact on our bodies when it is believed and when it is allowed to change our state of heart—that is, our moods and character.[1]

Shad Helmstetter, PhD, was one of the first behavioral researchers to focus on the role of self-talk. He dramatically demonstrated the principles of it in his own life. In his research working with top athletes, he had studied the impact of self-talk and how people's thoughts influence their behavior and performance. He decided to experiment on himself and address his own challenges with excess weight.

Dr. Helmstetter created his own audiotape full of healthy messages about eating well and becoming more active. On the recording, he told himself such things as "I love exercise" and "I am in control of my eating and enjoy healthy foods." Each morning as he shaved at his bathroom sink, he would play his tape on a cassette player.

Over the course of ten and a half weeks, he shed thirty-eight pounds. Interestingly, his wife, who was getting ready at the other sink, lost twenty-five pounds, and it wasn't even her tape![2] Dr. Helmstetter proved for himself the truth that the most dominant thought will ultimately drive behavior.

Simple Steps to Change Your Habits and Your Life

To realize the same kind of change, our minds require daily doses of positive self-talk. Changing our minds requires a consistent supply of powerful messages bombarding our neurons. When we don't choose to infuse transforming truths into our minds, we passively surrender control to the lies we believe or the negative influences of the world.

These four simple steps, a recap of what we've learned, will help you get started immediately on transforming your mind, habits, and life:

1. Identify the lies you believe.
2. Take unhealthy thoughts captive.
3. Replace lies with truth.
4. Practice healthy self-talk daily.

Step 1: Identify the Lies You Believe

It's important to notice and acknowledge the negative thoughts at the root of your unhealthy habits or other behaviors. We (Danna and Robyn) call them lies.

Sometimes people are not keenly aware of the lies because they're deep-seated and not always expressed in words. One of the easiest ways for you to recognize unhealthy thoughts is to identify the habits and behaviors that are holding you back. For example:

Habit or Behavior to Change	Lies You Believe
giving in to sweet cravings every day	*I deserve this sweet treat*
eating too much at a meal	*I have no self-control*
living a sedentary lifestyle	*I am lazy and have no energy*

Spend a few minutes thinking about why you chose this book. Then write down the habits and behaviors you want to change and record what you suspect are the lies that may be driving those behaviors.

Behavior to Change	Rationalization/Lie

Your strong negative habits are being pushed by strong negative thoughts. As you become more mindful of your thought life, you'll begin to better understand your underlying thoughts.

Behind all your negative emotions, there is an underlying thought. Ask yourself, *What does this feeling say about what I think?* If you're anxious, you are probably thinking a lot of anxious thoughts. If you are chronically discontent, you are likely dwelling on what you don't have rather than what you do have. There is a strong thought related to those persistent emotions, and it's like a deep rut in your neural pathway. In some cases, it's become a superhighway in your brain.

> Whatever is true, whatever is noble, whatever is right, whatever is pure, whatever is lovely, whatever is admirable—if anything is excellent or praiseworthy—think about such things.
>
> —Philippians 4:8

The good news is that persistent *positive* and delightful emotions are working for you in a beneficial way. When we dwell on positive things with an attitude of gratitude, emotions that enrich our lives follow!

To become more aware of your negative thinking, record your thoughts and feelings in a notebook. Use your smartphone alarm to nudge you periodically throughout the day to perform a quick reality check on your thinking. Document any negative self-talk, and take a few moments to replace those thoughts with a new message.

Step 2: Take Unhealthy Thoughts Captive

As you begin to identify the most dominant lies you believe, you will be more aware of when they pop into your mind or when they are driving you toward undesirable behavior. Your task is to switch focus immediately. One strategy is to ask God for the strength to stop dwelling on the negative. We call this *taking our thoughts captive.*

Try to recognize your unhealthy thoughts quickly and refuse to dwell on them. Imagine each is an ugly cockroach that you squash with the heel of your shoe. You have much more control than you realize, and this control will strengthen each day as you move through these steps on a regular basis.

Periodically review the notes you make in your thought notebook and ask yourself these questions:

- *What are the persistent unhealthy messages I repeat most often?*
- *What is the common theme?*
- *What unpleasant emotions do I experience frequently?*
- *What do these emotions say about my underlying thoughts?*

Write these questions and your answers in your notebook. Refer to them often until you are clear which thoughts need erasing. When they come to the surface of your conscious mind, take them captive immediately. See these emotions as flashing yellow lights alerting you to be cautious before they prompt you to action.

Step 3: Replace Lies with Truth

Finding the right healthy messages to replace your lies is essential to your success. For us, Scripture is a great place to start.

In addition, simple positive statements that counteract your specific challenges are also useful. Using your thought notebook, record the healthy statements you have chosen to counteract the lies you've believed. Add to this list or modify your statements as you become more self-aware.

- Whether you eat or drink or whatever you do, do it all for the glory of God. (1 Corinthians 10:31)
- Present your bodies as a living sacrifice, holy and acceptable to God, which is your spiritual worship. (Romans 12:1, ESV)
- I can do all things through him who strengthens me. (Philippians 4:13, ESV)
- I have great self-control and desire a lean, healthy body more than satisfying my taste buds with unhealthy foods.
- I eat only when I am hungry, and I am easily satisfied.

Listening to healthy self-talk audio recordings is an effective and simple way to transform our minds. For twenty-five years, Danna has used CD and digital recordings she created to help her clients and readers change their minds and habits. And more recently, we created a recording specifically for anyone following the Eat, Live, Thrive Diet. It's woven with Scripture and has healthy messages related to all three phases of the diet. You can find our recordings in both CD and MP3 formats at our web store, which can be found at LeanHealthyAgeless.com and EatLiveThriveDiet.com.

Step 4: Practice Healthy Self-Talk Daily

Fortunately, changing your mind is a simple process. However, it does take consistent effort. Identifying and writing down healthy self-talk is not enough. To make those messages take root, you need to repeat them often until new dominant thoughts form. If you persist over the weeks and months ahead, you will be pleasantly rewarded with a new level of motivation and self-discipline that drives you toward your best health and body.

This process happens in two stages. The *first stage* is what we call "top-of-the-mind awareness."

By practicing your new self-talk several times a day, you bring these messages into your conscious mind. Like a song that repeats itself in your mind all day long—even if you wish it wouldn't—your new self-talk will start to pop into your thoughts automatically.

Saying your self-talk messages out loud will enhance and speed up the process. Ideally, make your final thoughts for the day intentional and productive. Write down your new, healthy statements on index cards and keep them on your bedside table. Read these statements every night, or listen to a healthy self-talk recording just before you go to sleep.

The *second and most important stage* takes much longer. It is the process of physiologically changing your neural pathways. This doesn't even begin to take place for about twenty-one days. As you build the foundation of a healthy mind-set, your new messages eventually become dominant. In a few weeks, you may notice subtle changes in your attitude, emotions, and behavior. It gets easier to say no to your impulses.

When you notice improvement, don't stop repeating your healthy statements. We've been hearing old messages for many years and need to reinforce our new thoughts long after we start to experience the positive changes. When you go to the dentist to have a decayed tooth filled and are cavity free, you don't stop brushing your teeth. Your new healthy self-talk is a daily habit you need to practice to keep a "cavity-free" brain for the rest of your life!

Trigger Talk

A useful technique that will prompt you to repeat your customized self-talk several times each day is called trigger talk. This is how it works: Identify an activity you engage in one or more times each day. For example, every time you start your car or look at your watch, repeat your scripture or new statement. Use these events as triggers to remind you to repeat your new messages.

We call one of our favorite triggers "potty talk." Really! While some of us think of potty talk as swearing by an adult, we think of it as using our time in the bathroom as a trigger to change our thinking—"talking" to ourselves on the potty. It's the ultimate multitasking opportunity!

Another easy way to remind yourself to practice healthy self-talk is to put a rubber band around your toothbrush. You will notice the band, which will trigger you to silently say your top three or four statements during the minute or two you are brushing your teeth every morning and evening.

In our high-tech age, you can use electronics to trigger you. We set our smartphones to beep at us during the day when we want to memorize a new scripture or work on a new mental habit.

Just imagine how your focus in life would change if three times a day you were triggered to say or think statements such as these:

- I choose to honor God with my body. I know that his power is within me and will ask him for help in dealing with temptation and changing my lifestyle.
- I am an ageless woman, full of vitality and health because I choose to nurture myself well every day in how I eat, live, and thrive.

Find creative ways to remind yourself to use your trigger until you get into the trigger habit. You can tape your messages on the inside of your medicine cabinet, refrigerator door, or cupboard. You could put a Post-it note on your steering wheel. Do whatever it takes to remind yourself of your new activity.

The techniques used to change your thinking are simple. Doing them *consistently* is the challenge. We are creatures of habit, and we seem to forget what we've decided to do.

You will know that your trigger talk has become permanent when two things occur. First, your mind will automatically focus on that specific statement or scripture whenever you experience the trigger. Have you ever heard an old song and immediately remembered a time or place in your life? That's because the song is a powerful trigger associated with that experience.

The second thing that will validate the effectiveness of your trigger talk is that your feelings and behavior will start to change. Because your mind believes what you tell it most often, your behavior and feelings will reflect that new belief. The challenge is to practice long enough for those changes to take place.

Before choosing to adopt a new trend for health and weight loss, consider the upsides and downsides equally.

—DANNA AND ROBYN

Before we begin our in-depth discussion of the guidelines and phases of the Eat, Live, Thrive Diet, as well as the foods you'll be eating, we'd like to familiarize you with two very popular dieting trends that are said to significantly enhance your body's fat-burning potential.

The first—intermittent fasting—is focused exclusively on *when* and *how often* you eat. The second, ketogenic dieting, is focused on depleting your carbohydrate levels to the point that your body switches to a totally different metabolic process, with the main objective of burning fat rapidly. Both methods are also said to provide other health benefits.

Why should you know this? You may be told that these methods are the ultimate fat-burning strategies. That can be seductive! They are very effective, but the truth is, they come with risks and challenges.

We believe that the Eat, Live, Thrive approach we've designed is much more enjoyable and less restrictive than following only intermittent fasting or a ketogenic diet. The ELT approach also supports a more sustainable lifestyle, while reaping many of the same benefits for health and weight loss. We'll teach you our ELT strategies in the next chapter.

Your Body, a Survival Machine

Your body is not particularly concerned that you are storing more fat than you feel is desirable. In fact, it feels *more* secure when you are well stocked! But when you make drastic changes to how, what, and when you eat, your body gets worried and works hard to correct what it sees as a threat or stress.

According to Dr. Will Cole, a functional-medicine practitioner, women are more sensitive than men to intermittent fasting because of our unique body chemistry, and it could affect our metabolism and (for younger women) fertility.[1] Additionally, some experts are concerned with the stress that fasting can put on the adrenal glands. This not only pushes the body back into a fat-storing mode but also can cause undue fatigue or even exhaustion.

One of the body's first responses to stress is to release stress hormones, including cortisol. If this happens day after day, you can overwork your adrenal glands. Rather than feelings of high energy and well-being, exhaustion results. And in extreme cases, medical intervention may be needed. Therefore, it is very important—especially as a woman—to gently transition your body into a new eating schedule, which we will discuss shortly.

This is one reason we don't advise jumping into a 16/8 fasting-and-eating schedule too quickly. Many experts—including our nutrition adviser, Patti Milligan—believe that women do much better when they allow their bodies to slowly adapt to their ideal schedules.

This is especially true for those struggling with blood-sugar control. If your body is not accustomed to being in a fasting state for more than ten hours, a jump to sixteen hours could trigger a cortisol stress response. It is also essential to ask your physician if any lifestyle changes—especially increasing fasting windows—would affect any medications you are taking.

Understanding Your Body's Energy Pantry

Before we discuss the pros and cons of the two diet trends, it is helpful to understand the fuel sources that your body has available and also how you can nudge your body into becoming more metabolically adaptable with only a minimal amount of stress.

If your kitchen pantry, refrigerator, and freezer were overflowing with food, you'd most likely be delighted. But when it comes to our bodies, we sigh in frustration at the stored fuel that readily accumulates within our fat cells.

That ever-expanding adipose tissue is not the only source of fuel in our bodies' energy pantries. We have two other fuel sources. One we use every day unless it's been completely depleted; the other is a source of fuel we should use only under the direst of circumstances.

Understanding all this will help you better imagine what's going on inside your body so you can gently prod it into trusting you as you become a better fat-burning machine.

Your Carb Cupboards

Carbohydrates are your body's preferred fuel source. Your body converts both complex and simple carbohydrates to glucose so that it can fuel every cell in your body. After your body converts and burns all the carbohydrates from your most recent meal or snack, your cells turn their attention to your "carb cupboards," where carbs are stored in the form of glycogen in muscle tissue and the liver. This form of fuel is easy for the body to access.

The average woman holds about 2,000 calories of stored glycogen.[2] So what happens when your carb cupboards are totally full? Your body turns those excess carbohydrate calories into fat and stores them in your next fuel cupboard.

Also, most mature women who struggle with excess weight are insulin resistant too. If this is true for you, it means that your body does not adequately allow glucose into its cells for energy. Because you cannot survive with excess glucose in your bloodstream, your body goes into a protective mode and quickly converts these homeless carbohydrates into fat and stores them. *Oy vey.* That is the last thing you need! Stay tuned because there are many positive solutions to help prevent this from occurring.

Your Fat Cupboards

We've all seen evidence of the human body's almost unlimited capacity to store fat. Unlike our muscles' and livers' limited capacity, our fat cells expand to meet the storage need.

When excess calories are not burned, they are converted via a process called lipogenesis and stored as fat in fat cells. In times of famine, fat stores can fuel the body for weeks or even months. That need rarely arises outside developing countries. Instead, we drag around our extra fuel tanks and wish we could get our bodies to access those energy sources more readily. Well, we can! That's just one of the important benefits of adding short-term fasting into our long-term lifestyles.

Your Protein Cupboards

Let's look at our last fuel source, protein. Our bodies can and do convert our dietary protein into glucose for energy when necessary. However, stored protein in the form of muscle or organ tissue is accessed only under the direst of circumstances.

Fortunately, our bodies have great resources in place for times of fasting and even starvation that create a protein-sparing protection. God designed our metabolisms to protect our vital organs and muscles—which are mostly composed of protein—from being used as fuel. This alternate metabolic pathway that spares protein and uses fat for energy is called ketosis, and we'll discuss this more later in this chapter.

Intermittent Fasting

Let's first look at intermittent fasting, which the Eat, Live, Thrive approach does actually utilize to some degree. Practitioners of intermittent fasting claim that the benefits are weight loss, vitality, anti-aging, and disease prevention.

We understand that the concept of a fast does not appeal to many. You may immediately picture yourself feeling hungry or deprived. You may wonder, *Will my blood sugar tank? Will I be so fuzzy brained that I'll forget why I walked into the room?* (Not that most of us don't do that anyway!)

However, most women are surprised by how easy it is to make short-term fasting a regular component of their weekly lifestyle when they follow our guidelines and tips. After coaching thousands of women, we have learned that a simple lifestyle change in regard to fasting can make it easier for mature women to reach their health and weight-loss goals. We'll guide you through it.

Intermittent Fasting Is Nothing New

Intermittent fasting is not so much a new practice but rather the resurgence of an abandoned one. If we were to peek back in time to almost any era other than the last one hundred years, we'd likely see that most people lived this way naturally.

> The truth is that humans have been fasting for thousands of years. Modern research is playing catch-up, to understand why the health benefits are so impressive.
>
> —Cyrus Khambatta, PhD

Modern people think that their current lifestyles are normal, but actually they are further from "true normal" than most of us realize. As a culture, Americans eat more calories with fewer nutrients and live more sedentary lives than ever before. Perhaps we can learn some important lessons and be motivated by women of earlier times.

With that in mind, let's take a quick imaginary journey to a time when life was much simpler and lifestyles were much different . . .

Whoosh. You've just been transported to mid-nineteenth-century America. And like the majority of the population at the time, you live on a farm. Yep, this will probably be the new normal for you, girl!

As a farm woman, you get up at the crack of dawn (or earlier) each day and tend to various chores before you even think about breakfast. You never go to the gym or take more than a leisurely walk. The foods you eat are not found in freezer bags, boxes, cans, or bottles, either. You make most meals from the food you grow or from the items you get from other farmers. You are so active that you burn close to 3,000 calories per day and you eat that many calories a day as well. Woo-hoo!

But don't get too excited if you love potato chips or crackers or cookies. Those foods have to be made from scratch, and you rarely have the time or money for such indulgences. Yes, bread is a core part of your diet, but when it comes to treats, an occasional fresh apple pie on a weekend is the most you'll see—and you'll be lucky if you get more than a nibble with all those hungry mouths to feed.

While you do indeed eat much more food than your future self, you also eat it in a shorter window of time. It's likely that the average farm woman had an eating window of approximately eight to twelve hours per day and then fasted for twelve to sixteen hours as a normal part of her lifestyle.[3] For example, she may have eaten breakfast at 9 a.m. and then another meal around 2 p.m. If food was in sufficient supply, there may have been an early-evening snack. In this scenario, her eating window was about nine hours (from 9 a.m. to 6 p.m.) and her fasting window was fifteen hours (from 6 p.m. to 9 a.m.). However, she did not think about the fact that she was fasting; it was just her normal lifestyle.

So how does your lifestyle compare to the farm girl example? We know from working with thousands of women and from our own lives that many of us eat breakfast as early as 7 a.m. and take our last bites of food perhaps while watching television or reading in bed as late as 11 p.m. In this case, the eating window is sixteen hours and the fasting window only eight. That's a complete reversal from earlier times.

So what? you may be asking. *What does it matter* when *I eat as long as I burn all the calories I consume and maintain a reasonably healthy diet?*

We're glad you asked! There are many potential benefits to what has become known as intermittent fasting. At first glance, it may seem like a fad, but if not taken to excess, it has the potential to become a reasonable lifestyle habit that will serve us well. Intermittent fasting is not a specific diet but rather a strategic eating/fasting schedule that can be combined with any nutritional plan.

Benefits of Fasting

There are several reasons people lose weight with intermittent fasting. First, most end up eating fewer calories overall because of limiting their eating windows. This results in burning off some of their stored fat. However, there are others who tend to overeat after breaking their fasts, and that certainly defeats the effort.

It's important to gather all the information you can and test yourself to see how you respond. Robyn finds fasting highly beneficial in toning down her hunger issue and tends to eat less when she fasts twelve to sixteen hours most days.

Fasting Adventures: Client Results

Danna and Robyn's intermittent fasting method has absolutely worked for me. I was always one who thought I needed to eat breakfast. I've found that by putting off eating until later, I tend to eat fewer carbs, and I also fill up faster when I do eat. Since beginning their three-phase lifestyle plan, I've been very intentional about not eating after 6 p.m. and then not eating until around 10 or 11 a.m. the next day. To date, I have lost almost twenty-five pounds, and I've also lost my insatiable hunger! I allow myself healthy snacks when I am hungry, and I always have a nice dinner with my family.

—Sheila

This type of short-term fasting has been a game changer for me. I first heard about this in August during a coaching call with Danna and Robyn. Having just started their diet plan, I was intrigued and tried fasting that day. I had immediate results—not only weight loss, but my energy levels increased and I was thinking more clearly. Since August, I've lost eighteen pounds and fourteen inches—seven off my waist and seven off my hips and abdomen. My energy levels are great. It feels like I've turned back the clock!

—Sandi

I've been doing a form of intermittent fasting for years. I started to get rid of stubborn pounds when I was close to my goal weight. More than weight loss, I notice more mental clarity and a lot of energy before I start eating for the day.

—Tracey

As we mentioned earlier, a large percentage of mature women who struggle with weight loss have some level of insulin resistance. This makes it very difficult for them to lose weight and puts them at much higher risk of becoming diabetic. When insulin is present, the body does not burn fat effectively. However, during a fasting state, insulin production stops because no food is present, and this facilitates both fat burning and blood-sugar balance. That's why we believe some types of short-term fasting are highly effective for women over forty-five.

During fasting, the body initiates important cellular-repair processes, such as removing waste material from cells. This is known as autophagy, and it creates positive changes in several genes and molecules related to longevity and protection against disease.

Another great benefit (especially for mature women) is that fasting can positively influence glucose regulation. This is especially relevant because so many women are treading dangerously close to becoming diabetic.

With a doctorate in nutritional biochemistry, Cyrus Khambatta has dedicated his adult life to understanding fasting and its benefits. He was diagnosed with type 1 diabetes at the age of twenty-two, and as a result switched his college major and acquired his doctorate in nutrition because of his passion for this subject. He says,

> As far as glucose metabolism is concerned, intermittent fasting is an absolute goldmine. Intermittent fasting is an incredibly powerful tool for normalizing glucose and improving glucose variability. Apart from exercise, intermittent fasting is the most powerful natural insulin sensitizer known to man.
>
> The specific effects of intermittent fasting on diabetes are listed here:
> - Reduced fasting blood glucose
> - Reduced post-prandial (after meal) blood glucose
> - Reduced glucose variability
> - Increased insulin sensitivity[4]

Many experts believe that in addition to what we've already mentioned, there are additional benefits to intermittent fasting, such as
- reduction of oxidative stress and inflammation in the body
- protection against several diseases, including cancer and Alzheimer's disease[5]
- cellular rest and regeneration as organs get a break from metabolism

Anecdotally, we (Danna and Robyn) have discovered for both ourselves and our clients other, more subjective benefits. These include

- greater energy
- improved mental focus
- sharper memory
- better mood
- decreased hunger

I (Robyn) have been practicing short-term fasting—no fewer than twelve hours per day but often more—for about four years, and it greatly diminishes my insatiable appetite.

Bonus: Possible Breast Cancer Prevention

Our personal naturopathic medical doctor and adviser for this book, Dr. Mark Stengler,[6] pointed out an important study that gives women one more motivation for adding short-term fasting to their lifestyles.

In 2016, researchers studied approximately 2,400 women with early-stage breast cancer and determined that women who extended their nightly fasting window to at least thirteen hours could reduce the risk of cancer recurrence. In contrast, those who fasted fewer than thirteen hours had a 36 percent higher risk for disease recurrence.[7]

Fasting Options

For most of you, fasting will be no more than twelve to sixteen hours. You don't need to go a full day without food to reap the benefits of fasting. We'll offer you a variation of common intermittent-fasting practices, which we call the ELT Eating Cycle. We believe that it can improve both your health and weight-loss results. However, it is important to note that it is not for everyone. Listen to your body and consult with your health-care professional to be sure it is appropriate for you.

We'll describe our method in detail in the next chapter. Meanwhile, it may be helpful to understand what many popular intermittent-fasting programs look like. Most experts consider a true intermittent fast to be from as few as fourteen hours to a maximum of thirty-six hours. The most popular programs tend to encourage fasting from twenty to thirty-six hours a few times per week. Some allow up to 500 calories during a twenty-four-hour fasting period. Many recommend never doing an extended fast like this on consecutive days. These types of fasting programs work especially well for men.

For many mature women, these more intense protocols can lead to some challenges we'll discuss shortly. You may be willing to do a twenty-four-hour fast occasionally for spiritual reasons—a topic we'll address later—but do you want that to be a part of your permanent weekly lifestyle? Not so much! And twenty-four- to thirty-six-hour fasts take a lot of willpower and can be stressful to the body in various ways.

While many of the benefits of intermittent fasting have been studied with longer fasting periods, we believe there are incremental benefits for those choosing much shorter fasting windows. This is what Dr. Joseph Mercola—a popular osteopathic physician, web blogger, author, and alternative-medicine proponent—says:

> Simply restricting your daily eating to a narrower window of time of say 6–8 hours, you can reap the benefits without the suffering. This equates to 16–18 hours worth of fasting each and every day—enough to get your body to shift into fat-burning mode.[8]

Whereas constant eating may lead to metabolic exhaustion and health consequences such as weight gain, studies suggest that our bodies may benefit from the break they receive while fasting. This is great news! By simply narrowing our daily eating windows to eight hours per day, we can improve our health and stay leaner.

Several studies have investigated the effects of a 16/8 fasting-and-eating regimen. One review published in the journal *Behavioral Sciences* in early 2017 looked at recent studies comparing the weight-loss effects of intermittent fasting and low-calorie diets and concluded that the fasting approach appeared to be as effective as low-calorie diets at reducing body weight in obese and overweight people.[9]

Ketogenic Diets

It's likely you've been hearing the buzz about ketogenic diets for quite some time. They were introduced in the 1920s, when it was discovered that a keto diet greatly reduced seizures in epileptics, especially children.[10] Ketosis became best known as a weight-loss method when Dr. Robert Atkins published his book *Dr. Atkins' Diet Revolution* in 1972. It achieved a higher level of exposure and acclaim with his best-selling updated version, *Dr. Atkins' New Diet Revolution,* in 1992.

People burned fat. People lost weight. People rebounded. Despite all the bioengineered low-carb foods, many people could not sustain the diet or their weight loss. Nevertheless, here we go again.

Today, for the most part, there seems to be a healthier emphasis on the quality and ratio of foods. In the past, people were told to eat any, and as many, proteins or fats they desired. While the fat-burning chemistry still worked, the health risks were evident. Too much protein creates a very heavy workload on the body. And unhealthy fats produce another list of potential health traps.

> **Whether you eat or drink or whatever you do, do it all for the glory of God.**
>
> —1 Corinthians 10:31

Many practitioners, including Dr. Joseph Mercola, who promote a healthier ketogenic approach recommend a diet that is at least 70 percent healthy fats (such as olive or coconut oil), less than 10 percent quality proteins (such as organic poultry or grass-fed beef), with the remaining 30 percent focused on low-glycemic vegetables. This means that you'll need to be very creative and find ways to add lots of healthy fats to your veggies. And, it also means you'll be removing veggies such as peas, carrots, and potatoes from your diet.

There Are Downsides

Even with these positive changes to the keto diet, it is our opinion there are still two major downsides: first, the diet is hard to sustain for most people; second, it lacks dietary balance.

We believe our ELT Diet and Lifestyle Plan and ELT Eating Cycle methods can provide you with many of the benefits of a ketogenic diet without the rigorous requirements needed to stay in full compliance.

Also, if God designed this ketogenic pathway to save our lives in times of famine and potential starvation, perhaps there is a relevant spiritual question we should ask: Do you believe that tricking your body into thinking it is starving so you can burn off excess fat is being a good steward of your health? Only you can answer that for yourself. We place no judgment!

Please don't misinterpret what we are saying. We acknowledge that you *can* eat quite healthily on a well-thought-out keto diet—for a while. Yes, you are likely to burn fat faster than you ever have before. However, it is up to you to determine if it is a wise approach from both a physical and a spiritual perspective. While there are some scientifically proven benefits beyond fat burning, do those justify going to the extreme of full-blown ketosis? Will this be a healthy long-term approach for you?

On the *Harvard Health Blog,* Dr. Marcelo Campos has this to say about ketogenic diets:

A ketogenic diet could be an interesting alternative to treat certain conditions, and may accelerate weight loss. But it is hard to follow and it can be heavy on red meat and other fatty, processed, and salty foods that are notoriously unhealthy. We also do not know much about its long-term effects, probably because it's so hard to stick with that people can't eat this way for a long time. It is also important to remember that "yo-yo diets" that lead to rapid weight loss fluctuation are associated with increased mortality. Instead of engaging in the next popular diet that would last only a few weeks to months (for most people that includes a ketogenic diet), try to embrace change that is sustainable over the long term.[11]

If you choose to use a keto approach for a time on your weight-loss journey, we encourage you to use our plan as your transition back to a more sustainable long-term eating plan. We will teach you how to rotate through each phase of our diet periodically throughout each year to gain and maintain a lean and healthy body no matter your age. It *is* possible!

PART 2

THE PLAN

Limiting eating to fewer hours each day frees your body up from the hard work of digestion and gives it more time to replenish and promote agelessness.

—Danna and Robyn

The female body is a touchy machine. She's highly reactive to change and constantly seeking assurance that she is not being overstressed. She responds to a gentle nudge much more positively than an aggressive push. When she feels secure, she purrs like a well-tuned Ferrari.

In calorie restriction, many studies have concluded that losing weight slowly protects the metabolism. For many women, creating a calorie deficit of greater than 500 calories per day can work against her as the body interprets it as a threat for survival. When this happens, the metabolism declines, weight loss halts, and the Ferrari has now become an energy-efficient (fat-hoarding) Prius.

We believe the same can be true when adding fasting into your lifestyle. A gradual approach gives your body time to adapt. It also provides you with a mental and emotional transition that allows you to hone your self-discipline and willpower capabilities. We also hope that you are already implementing healthy self-talk strategies into your daily lifestyle.

Ease on Down the Road

It's best to start your short-term Eat, Live, Thrive Eating Cycle right where you live. To do that, you need to tune in to your usual eating patterns:

- What time do you normally eat your last meal of the day?
- What time do you eat your last snack or even nibble of food for the day?
- What time do you wake up in the morning?
- What time do you normally eat your first meal?

Fasting Step 1

The first goal we recommend is to work toward twelve hours fasting and twelve hours eating as your new normal (remember the farm woman from the previous chapter!). We call this the 12/12 cycle.

As an example, if you stop eating at eight at night, you will not eat again until at least eight the next morning. What was once the normal pattern for most women in the past can become your new normal.

The single biggest demand on the human body is digestion. Giving your body a break from processing food is healthy on many levels and there are anti-aging benefits too. Instead of your gut working on getting your last kernel of popcorn digested and into the proper storage cupboard, there are extra resources available to regenerate other cells throughout your body as you sleep.

One of the best ways to supersize this lifestyle strategy is to take your last bite of food or sip of caloric beverage three hours before you go to bed. This new habit keeps you out of that weight-gaining danger zone—the time when you eat calories and carbs you don't truly need. Does anyone *need* a bowl of ice cream to fuel up before sleeping?

Give this 12/12 cycle a try right away. It is a very easy new habit to add and will serve you well for life.

Sleep on This

As you stop eating at an earlier time, go to bed and consider all the positive things that are happening on a cellular level as the hours pass. Glycogen levels (your carb cupboards) are slowly emptying. At eight to twelve hours, your body begins to shift to using more fat as a fuel source by producing ketones, which also can increase energy, balance blood sugar, and improve satiety.

Isn't it great to get so much done while you're sleeping? You go, girl!

Speaking of sleep, did you know that many well-conducted studies have validated that getting at least seven hours of good-quality sleep each night is essential for weight loss, not to mention an excellent anti-aging strategy? We give you some great sleeping tips in chapter 13.

Hitting the Wall Before Twelve Hours?

If you find yourself hitting the wall (feeling extra hungry, light headed, shaky), you may have some blood-sugar instability and will need to ease into the first fasting step more slowly.

For example, if you're a gal who takes her last bite of ice cream (be it ever so small) at 10 p.m. before hitting the sack and usually eats breakfast at 7 a.m., you've been living a 9/15 fasting-and-eating cycle. Start by quitting eating earlier in the evening; however, go ahead and break your fast as soon as you feel the need. In this example, you stop eating at 8 p.m. and then resume perhaps at 7 a.m.—an eleven-hour fast. Just keep working at it until you can do 12/12 consistently with your only exception being special occasions and travel.

When you begin the Elimination Phase of our diet, this new normal becomes even easier because your meals and snacks are lower in starchy carbohydrates and higher in protein, fat, and fiber. This will bring you greater blood-sugar stability, satiety, and energy.

Fasting Step 2

To gain the extra benefits of fasting—including extended fat burning, production of ketones for brain health and energy, and health rewards such as improved insulin response and decreased inflammation—you may want to consider increasing the length of your fast a few times during the week.

You can slowly work up to a fourteen- or sixteen-hour fast some days. Tune in to your body and be aware of your response to fasting. Some people can jump right into a 16/8 cycle and realize immediate benefits and feel great. Others will need to take it very slowly and may never extend beyond a 14/10 cycle. The key is to capture the benefits of fasting and avoid the downsides.

Because you won't know for sure if you're the "jump right in" kind of gal, we suggest you start increasing by one hour per day until you reach your ideal fasting/eating hours. Here's an example:

Day	Fasting Hours	Eating Hours
Monday	10	14
Tuesday	11	13
Wednesday	12	12
Thursday	13	11
Friday	12	12
Saturday	14	10
Sunday	12	12
Monday	15	9
Tuesday	12	12
Wednesday	16	8

If you can adapt to the 16/8 cycle without difficulty, you can continue using that level of fasting. We suggest that you do a 16/8 cycle no more than three days per week to ensure you are not overly taxing your body. Take note of the information on pages 54–55 about the liquids you can drink during your fasting cycle and what you can add to your coffee, tea, or sparkling water.

Many women love the benefits they realize with fasting and are motivated to fast up to sixteen hours most days. If you are one of those women, listen carefully to your body. There are various telltale signs that you may be pushing your fasting limit.

Our nutrition adviser, Patti Milligan, says that the number one reason women wake up in the middle of the night is a significant drop in blood sugar. (And you thought it was your weak bladder!) Low blood sugar can be the result of what you ate for your last meal or the result of your fasting efforts stressing your body. Fatigue can be another telling symptom.

Adrenal Burnout

Speaking of fatigue and stress, we mentioned this earlier and it bears repeating: one of the biggest downsides for women fasting regularly can be adrenal fatigue. Even without fasting, it is not uncommon for mature women to have some level of adrenal burnout.

The best way to know definitively is through blood work. However, there are also some common signs:

- difficulty waking up and getting out of bed in the morning
- needing coffee to wake up fully
- gaining weight, especially around the waist
- getting frequent colds or the flu
- increasing difficulty dealing with daily stresses
- feeling light headed after standing up quickly
- craving salty foods
- needing food for energy or to get rid of low-blood-sugar jitters
- lack of interest in sex
- being tired in the early evening but then having a second wind if staying up
- unexplained pain or tension in the upper back or neck
- if still having periods: heavy bleeding, PMS symptoms, moodiness, increased fatigued
- feeling better on weekends or vacation when demands are low
- heart palpitations
- low body temperature
- dry skin
- disrupted bowel function (diarrhea or constipation)

Unfortunately, many of these symptoms can be related to other physical challenges, such as problems with thyroid function. That is why it is always wise to get regular checkups and blood work done so you can get to the root cause of your symptoms.

I Deserve This! And Self-Control

A potential shortfall of fasting can be what we call rebound eating, which is more an emotional than a physical response. It happens when you rationalize your fasting hours as permission to throw caution to the wind during your eating cycle and end up eating more rather than fewer overall calories.

It is crucial to tune in to this mind-set and cut back on fasting if rebound eating becomes a challenge for you. Go into your fast with a plan of how you will not only break your fast but also eat for the remainder of your eating window.

There is a positive flip side when it comes to fasting. Many women learn for the first time just how much self-control they truly have. By using this new strength wisely and exerting the same discipline when choosing food during your eating cycle, you'll obtain excellent and sustained results. When you consistently practice our gentle ELT Eating Cycle, you will continue to reap the rewards of improved metabolic agility, which will promote fat burning, blood-sugar balance, and insulin sensitivity.

Advanced Fasting Options

If you respond very positively to the 16/8 cycle, you may decide periodically to fast for twenty to twenty-four hours, as Robyn does. Danna almost never does. You may choose to do this for the extended benefits of metabolic rest or even for spiritual reasons. As always, listen carefully to your body. Nurture it well.

Tips to Make Your Eat, Live, Thrive Eating Cycle Sustainable

Rewire Your Thought Process: Think of fasting as taking a break from eating rather than a period of deprivation. As you focus on all the benefits, you can see each extra hour as an opportunity to get healthier and leaner. Just don't take this positive thinking to an extreme!

Try Different Timing Options: It may take a week or more to discover which fasting and eating times work best for your body and schedule. Though we recommend eating the last meal of the day earlier and ceasing from eating three hours before you go to bed, there may be a different schedule that works better for your lifestyle.

(continued on the next page)

Be Flexible: If you decided to fast for sixteen hours and you're crashing at fourteen hours, break your fast early and try to increase your fasting hours more gradually. If you're under extra stress, a 12/12 cycle may be the most you can handle for a while. That's okay.

Stay Busy: It may seem counterintuitive, but the best plan is often to start your fast when you're busy, not on a day when you'll be sitting on the couch wanting to snack. One of the challenges of eating healthily is deciding what to eat and having the time to shop for or prepare those foods. By shortening your eating window, you don't experience so much decision fatigue and are therefore freed up to do other things.

Busy or not, you should avoid longer fasting days during a week when you have increased mental or physical demands. For example, don't fast for sixteen hours if you have a major business presentation or project that requires high-level attention. Once your body has adapted, a sixteen-hour fast may be a piece of cake for you. But you don't want to find out the hard way that you lose your mental focus at the fifteenth hour and cannot find the right words to speak coherently.

Exercise: Leading an active lifestyle is essential to being lean, healthy, and ageless. We'll address this topic in more detail in chapter 12. For most people, doing moderate-level exercise during the 12/12 cycle should be fine. However, if you exercise in the morning and find yourself losing energy or endurance, consider breaking your fast early with some natural sugar (fructose) found in a half serving of fruit such as half a banana. Or try a protein such as a few nuts or a hard-boiled egg.

Over time, your body will adjust to exercising in a fasting state. In fact, doing so can increase your fat-burning potential because your energy demand is so much higher during a workout. Ease into this routine slowly and do your easier workouts on longer fasting days to start. A brisk walk and lightweight workout will improve your circulation and may even make the last couple of hours of your fast easier.

Drink Plenty of Fluids: Staying well hydrated is essential for good health and will make fasting periods much easier. Water should be your primary drink, but you can get some of your hydration from tea, a small amount of coffee, and sparkling water.

Too much caffeine from coffee or tea can raise cortisol and create an insulin response, which may diminish your fat burning. Some studies show that decaffeinated coffee helps minimize hunger more than regular coffee. (We recommend choosing organic coffee and Swiss Water Process decafs.)

Many people like to add cream or milk to these beverages. You can do so in moderation if you keep the carbohydrates to less than 1 gram and don't exceed 25 total calories in a three-hour period. Use half-and-half, unsweetened coconut milk (not canned), or unsweetened almond milk. It bears mentioning that you will find coconut milk in two very different versions. The first can be found in boxes, cartons, or other types of containers and is a thin, milky liquid best for beverages and for use in some recipes. The second variety is found in cans and is a much thicker, richer type of product and is almost solid, much like sour cream. This canned version has more calories and fat, and we will specify when to use canned coconut milk in certain recipes. If not mentioned, use the thinner, liquid option.

Do not use milk, because it is higher in carbs. Our favorite almond milk is Califia Farms Toasted Coconut. It has only 22 calories for one half cup, which is enough to lighten three cups of beverages.

Herbal tea is always good for staying hydrated and not overusing caffeine. Warm bone broth is also very healthy and filling. Sparkling water is fine. You can squeeze a few drops of lemon or lime into your water. Adding mint or cucumbers can also give it a refreshing non-caloric flavor. Avoid all juices. And you didn't even want to ask about diet soda, right? Right!

Use Lovidia's Hunger-Control Formula: This cutting-edge hunger-control supplement can be a very effective tool to help you begin and sustain the ELT Eating Cycle component of our diet. It is all natural and doesn't have any stimulants.

In addition, some of the ingredients have been shown to support optimal blood-sugar balance. More importantly, the formula helps your gut communicate with your brain to tell it that you are fully satisfied. It has helped Robyn significantly with her huge hunger issue, and Danna finds it especially helpful for extending her intermittent fasting to sixteen or more hours some days. Lovidia is one of the supplements we feature on our website EatLiveThriveDiet.com.

The Elimination Phase

Jump-Starting Your Health and Weight Loss

My body, mind, and spirit responded beautifully to the Elimination Phase of this diet. I had not known just how good I could feel until I implemented Danna and Robyn's system.

—BLANCHE W.

We've finally reached the diet portion of the book! Maybe just saying the word *diet* makes you feel deprived. But if you understand its real meaning, you may relax a little. Patti Milligan reminded us that the Greek word we get *diet* from means "a way of living."[1] That can include not just how we eat but also the types of habits we regularly practice.

Technically, you are always on a diet, even when you feel completely out of control and the quality of your nutrition is less than ideal. In those times, we don't go around proclaiming, "I'm on a diet to see how much weight I can gain by eating unlimited sugar and junk food!" We just coast along until we're ready to choose a healthier approach and then we declare the new "diet" we've adopted.

Perhaps you could benefit from writing your own definition that can inspire a new attitude and behavior. Here's one that resonates with us:

I choose a lean, healthy, and thriving lifestyle by intentionally eating and living in ways that maximize my vitality, minimize my weight and risk of disease, and allow me to fully enjoy my life.

You'll notice that we include the word *choose*. You are the CEO of your body and lifestyle. You get to *choose* how you want to eat and live.

By choosing our Eat, Live, Thrive approach, you've made a profound decision to engage in a new lifestyle, and you will be given the opportunity to create a lasting way of life that is customized to your unique desires and needs. We'll coach you along the way so you can make wise choices and proceed at a pace that suits your current life situation.

To keep things simple for you, we've included a "Success Steps at a Glance" synopsis at the end of the chapter to help you review the Elimination Phase steps and make decisions that will support you best.

Our three-phase diet plan is very doable. Even in this first elimination phase, as you jump-start your weight loss, you can enjoy a wide variety of foods and never feel hungry.

Here's what some of our clients have experienced in the Elimination Phase:

This diet has recipes that taste delicious! This is not a diet where we're forced to suffer eating celery sticks or what I call "rabbit food." The recipes are also loved by my husband, who is not watching his weight! —Tracey

The Elimination Phase helped me seek out healthy meal and snack alternatives instead of reaching for the same bad choices. It also helped me discover foods that were inhibiting my weight loss. Some foods that are considered healthy I found were making me sick. Now I enjoy eating to feel better. —Sandi F.

Overview of the Elimination Phase

Ready to jump-start your health and weight loss? This phase will help you do just that. You'll notice new vitality from removing many of the problematic foods that cause weight gain and inflammation throughout your body. You'll likely experience benefits beyond weight loss, such as improved energy, fewer aches and pains, better sleep, and clearer skin.

The Elimination Phase will also prepare you for the next important phase, Discovery, in which you'll identify the specific food culprits sabotaging your efforts.

We'll show you some of the key foods to remove, and we'll encourage you to make some changes to the quality of those you choose from the approved list. For example, we believe most vegetable oils are wreaking havoc on our bodies, causing systemic inflammation and potential disease.

The quality of what we eat on a regular basis is more important than ever as we age because our bodies lose resilience, and the accumulation of additives, pesticides, hormones, antibiotics, and genetically modified foods takes a toll. We'll discuss this topic in more depth in chapter 10. In the meantime, we'll provide some key nutritional recommendations in this chapter.

Three Levels to Choose From

We realize that getting started is the most important step. Just doing *something* is far better than waiting for the perfect time—some future tomorrow—to get going. After all, when it comes to dieting, tomorrow almost never arrives. Therefore, we've created three levels for you to choose from when participating in this phase. Level 3 will produce the most dramatic results. However, it takes a bit more planning, preparation, and effort. That's why we give you two options that allow you an easier transition.

All three levels can produce excellent results. We *do* hope that you will give Level 3 a spin at least once a year, even if it's not where you decide to start. It is ideal if you can do a Level 3 Elimination Phase four times a year, with each changing season. It's a perfect reset and cleansing time that gives you a fresh health boost, like a periodic spring cleaning for your body! It also gives you a chance to more fully realize how much better your body does with the elimination of certain foods.

The chart on the following page gives you, at a glance, which foods we recommend you eliminate at each of the three levels.

After your first fourteen-day elimination, you also can, on a monthly basis, do a seven-day elimination reboot. It's an opportunity to reevaluate any foods you are still uncertain about. We'll address this more in the Lifestyle Phase (see chapter 9).

Progress, Not Perfection

Once you decide whether you're going to tackle Level 1, 2, or 3, do your best to stay on the eating plan as closely as possible. But if a slipup happens, don't let that deter you. This is a good time to toss out any all-or-nothing attitudes and replace them with a reset-and-regroup mentality that gets you back on track quickly. The long-term objective is progress, not perfection.

Regardless of your specific goal, changing long-standing habits takes time. We've seen tons of women be amazed by how much can be accomplished in fourteen days. Obviously, the journey cannot stop there. We all know how easy it is to gain back the weight we've lost. Therefore, decide right now to participate in all three phases of this diet so you can realize long-term success!

You'll spend most of your life in Phase 3, the Lifestyle Phase. However, you'll get your best long-term results using all three phases (Elimination, Discovery, and Lifestyle) periodically as needed to realize your ideal weight and lock in your lifestyle habits.

The Elimination Phase At a Glance		
LEVEL 1	**LEVEL 2**	**LEVEL 3**
Eliminate: all grains all sugar* **For better results, eliminate:** alcohol artificial sweeteners potatoes, white	**Eliminate:** additives all grains all sugar* artificial sweeteners beans/legumes cold cuts cured meats dairy nuts preservatives vegetable oils** **For better results, eliminate:** alcohol potatoes, white	**Eliminate:** all grains all sugar* additives alcohol artificial sweeteners beans/legumes caffeinated beverages cold cuts cured meats dairy eggs nuts potatoes, white preservatives shellfish soy vegetable oils** **For detox, add:** body brushing box breathing cleansing drink cranberry drink supplements
* 1 tablespoon honey or maple syrup per day is allowed	* 1 tablespoon honey or maple syrup per day is allowed ** use avocado, olive, or coconut oil instead	* 1 tablespoon honey or maple syrup per day is allowed ** use avocado, olive, or coconut oil instead

Understanding the Guidelines and Troublesome Foods

Note that there are overlapping guidelines for each level. For the most part, we will detail the changes (additions and deletions) for Levels 2 and 3 when we describe them. Before we begin with Level 1, we want you to see the full list of troublesome foods that could be derailing your weight loss and causing you various unwanted symptoms:

- beans and legumes
- dairy
- eggs
- flours made with grains or nuts
- grains (to include corn and quinoa)
- nuts
- soy
- sugar

At some point, you will want to be sure you test all these foods. Most women are not aware of their personal food culprits.

Level 1 Guidelines

Level 1 is designed for the busy, overwhelmed, or apprehensive woman who needs a very simple and minimally restrictive starting point. In this level, we focus on eliminating two food types that are the main culprits at the core of the obesity epidemic: sugar and grains. If you eliminate these foods, you *will* realize results.

We recommend that you follow this plan for a full fourteen days before beginning the Discovery Phase. The list of eliminated foods is rather short, as you can see. We've also included a list of preferred foods to make part of your diet during the Elimination Phase. As you continue your nutrition journey, adding healthier options will enhance your overall wellness, longevity, and outward beauty.

Foods to Eliminate
- sugar and all foods containing processed sugar*
- all grains: barley, buckwheat, corn, couscous, flours made from grains, oats, quinoa, rice, rye, wheat.

* 1 tablespoon of raw, organic honey or pure maple syrup is allowed each day and best enjoyed in our grain-free recipes.

Foods to Include

The Elimination Phase isn't all about taking food out of your life. This long list of preferred food is full of possibilities!

Proteins

- beef
- eggs
- fish
- lamb
- pork
- poultry
- tofu and tempeh
- whey protein powder, high quality

Produce

- avocados
- beans (½ cup, 2 times per week)
- fruits (3 servings per day, maximum)
- vegetables (4–6 servings per day, minimum)
- potatoes, sweet (½ cup, 2-3 times per week)

Want Better Results in Level 1?

Also eliminating these foods and drinks will promote faster and more dramatic results:

- artificial sweeteners
- beer
- potatoes, white (including french fries and potato chips)
- spirits
- wine

We'll address the subject of alcoholic beverages in more detail in chapter 10.

Healthy Fats

- avocado oil
- butter
- coconut milk (canned, full-fat)
- extra-virgin coconut oil
- extra-virgin olive oil
- ghee (clarified butter)
- MCT (medium-chain triglyceride) oil
- nuts (¼ cup per day, maximum)
- sesame oil

Beverages and Liquids

- almond and coconut milk (unsweetened)
- bone broth (benefits on page 75)
- chicken broth, organic
- coffee and caffeinated tea (two 8-ounce cups per day)
- green tea
- herbal teas, iced or hot
- sparkling cranberry mocktail (see recipe on page 235)
- sparkling lemonade (see recipe on page 235)
- sparkling water, flavored optional (no artificial sweeteners)
- water—80 ounces per day (includes herbal tea)
- yerba mate tea

Seasoning

- cocoa powder, unsweetened
- fresh herbs
- sea salt and pepper
- spices, all

Condiments

- apple butter, unsweetened (1 tablespoon per day, maximum)
- apple cider vinegar
- horseradish

- hot sauces
- mustard
- red wine vinegar

Optional Foods for Healthy Cooking
- coconut flour or shredded unsweetened coconut
- honey, raw (1 tablespoon per day, maximum)**
- pure maple syrup, unrefined and organic (1 tablespoon per day, maximum)**
- stevia, liquid lo han, pure monk fruit extract
- tapioca flour

** *Keep in mind that your total honey or syrup servings per day should not exceed 1 tablespoon. Ideally, divide the tablespoon into three 1-teaspoon servings within a four-hour period.*

Snack or Portable-Lunch Ideas
- cold chicken or turkey rolled around avocado slice
- eggs, hard-boiled
- grain-free English muffins (see recipe on page 188)
- raw veggies and fruit
- salmon or tuna patties (see recipe on page 207)
- tuna and celery (with lemon and olive oil)

Level 2 Guidelines

Level 2 is designed for the woman who is ready to commit to eliminating most troublesome foods, except for eggs and soy (which are eliminated in Level 3). This expanded elimination list can produce faster and more dramatic results than Level 1 and prepare you for a more extensive food discovery in Phase 2.

Foods to Eliminate
(Same as Level 1)
- sugar
- all grains: barley, buckwheat, corn, couscous, flour (all kinds except coconut), oats, quinoa, rice, rye, wheat.

(Additional Eliminations for Level 2)
- beans and legumes
- dairy
- nuts

(Additional Foods to Eliminate—for Health Purposes)
- artificial sweeteners of all kinds
- cold cuts and cured meats
- foods packaged with additives and preservatives
- vegetable oils (except olive and avocado)

Foods to Include
You may include all foods on the Level 1 list except beans, butter, and nuts.

Level 3 Guidelines

Are you ready to get the maximum results possible in the next fourteen days? Do you want to not only jump-start your weight loss but also improve your overall health by cleansing your body of toxins? If your answer is yes, then Level 3 is for you.

In this level, you will eliminate eggs, soy, caffeine, white potatoes, and alcohol, in addition to all the eliminated foods in Level 2. Although this level may seem extreme, it is only temporary and the benefits you may experience will be more than worth the effort.

Want Better Results in Level 2?

Also eliminating these foods and drinks will promote faster and more dramatic results:
- beer
- potatoes, white (including french fries and potato chips)
- spirits
- wine

Some women feel younger and more healthy than they have in decades:

Thanks to God for directing me to Danna and Robyn! For the past sixteen years, I have felt my hips getting stiffer and stiffer. Of course, I gained weight as well and was not able to exercise like I needed. I was diagnosed with hip bursitis and have had many types of physical therapy. I've also seen a number of specialists, and no one could identify the underlying reason for my continued pain and immobility.

I am a NEW person! I've lost twenty-two pounds, and the decrease in inflammation in my body after doing Phase 1 of the diet has allowed me to walk again with ease! I kid you not—my husband and I were both thinking I would need to use a walker in the very near future. Now I take only a low dose anti-inflammatory on occasion and I feel better than I have in years.

Thank you so much! —Melanie

In Level 3, you'll also add a few supplements and drinks that will promote gentle detoxification. And by the way, your body does experience some cleansing and detoxification during Level 1 and Level 2 because you are giving it a break from so many bothersome foods.

Here's a quick recap of all the foods you'll eliminate for Level 3:

Foods to Eliminate
(Same as Level 2)

- sugar
- all grains: barley, buckwheat, corn, couscous, flour (all kinds except coconut), oats, quinoa, rice, rye, wheat
- beans and legumes
- dairy
- nuts

(Additional Eliminations for Level 3)

- additives and preservatives
- alcoholic beverages (wine, beer, spirits)
- artificial sweeteners
- coffee and caffeinated beverages
- cold cuts and cured meats
- eggs (last 4 days)***
- potatoes, white

- shellfish
- soy
- vegetable oils (except olive and avocado)

*** *Eggs can be a hidden sensitivity for some women, yet they are also one of the best protein sources. Therefore, we will eliminate them only for the last four days of Level 3 so you can enjoy many of our grain-replacement recipes and other recipes. However, if you suspect you could have a sensitivity, we recommend you eliminate eggs from the beginning.*

Foods to Include

You may include all foods on the Level 1 list except eggs, tofu, tempeh, nuts, beans, butter, coffee, and caffeinated tea.

Gentle Detoxification

Don't worry—detoxification is not an aggressive experience that will send you running to the bathroom all day long. It is a gentle but very effective cleanse when you follow the additional components noted in this section. Also, any of these cleansing strategies can be added to Level 1 and Level 2 if desired.

From experience, we know there probably will be one or two cleansing elements that won't work for you. While it is ideal to follow Level 3 totally, don't let a specific component of the program deter you from participating. Do your best to follow all the protocols, but give yourself permission to modify if you must.

As already mentioned (but worth repeating), we encourage you to participate in this Level 3 option quarterly, at the change of every season, to give your body the support it needs to perform most efficiently. It will help you burn fat to the max, improve your immunity, and enhance your energy. This is how you can truly realize what it means to feel ageless.

> It's hard to believe how well the Elimination/Cleansing phase works. The recipes are so good and I feel better than I have in years.
>
> —Jackie

Cleansing components for Level 3 include:

1. ELT cleansing drink
2. cranberry drink
3. fiber supplements
4. other supplements
5. body brushing

Please consider all the recommendations in this section. However, if you choose not to follow them all, we've listed them in order of priority.

1. ELT Cleansing Drink

We suggest that you drink the ELT cleansing drink before every meal. Here's the recipe:

1 cup raw apple cider vinegar
1 cup fresh lemon juice
2 teaspoons cinnamon
1 ½ teaspoons ground ginger
Stevia, liquid lo han, or pure monk fruit extract to taste

Mix ingredients in a large jar or shaker bottle and shake well. Add 2 tablespoons of the mixture to 4 to 12 ounces of hot or cold water. Sweeten more if needed. (Makes 16 servings.)

Drink 5 to 10 minutes before meals. Though acidic in the mouth, this drink creates an alkaline environment in the body. Rinse your mouth with water after each dose to prevent damaging tooth enamel when taken frequently.

The ingredients within this drink support cleansing and weight loss, and they promote detoxification throughout your body:

- *Raw apple cider vinegar* is known for boosting the metabolism. The acetic acid may support the production of stomach acid, which aids the digestive process and helps increase the absorption of nutrients. It also helps grow the good bacteria (known as probiotics) in your gut. Probiotics help with the detoxification of your colon. Studies have also shown that taking one to two tablespoons before a meal may promote blood-sugar stability and help with satiety.
- *Fresh lemon juice* aids in the digestive process. The citric acid assists the body's natural cleansing system in flushing out toxins and supports immunity. The pectin fiber helps with appetite control by giving a feeling of fullness. Lemons also have a strong alkalinizing effect that brings balance to your body's pH level.
- *Cinnamon* has been shown to improve insulin sensitivity, help promote blood-sugar stability, and support healthy blood pressure. It also has anti-inflammatory properties.
- *Ginger* is highly anti-inflammatory and aids in digestion and detoxification.

As you can see, the first two ingredients are highly acidic. However, when taken on an empty stomach, they cause a systemic alkaline reaction (a good thing). The acids also stimulate your own digestive acids so they can go to work on your upcoming meal.

Many women who struggle with heartburn, acid reflux, and indigestion are quite surprised that this drink calms their symptoms. However, for those of you who have an extremely sensitive throat or esophagus, dilute as needed initially and then very gradually work toward full strength if possible. A few of you may not be able to tolerate it right now, but you may find that the elimination diet improves your gut health and you can tolerate it later.

2. Cranberry Drink

Unsweetened, pure cranberry juice has natural organic acids that help emulsify fatty deposits throughout your lymphatic system. This juice diminishes water retention, balances blood sugar, helps break down cellulite, and assists your liver and lymphatic system with the detoxification process.

To prepare the cranberry drink, dilute 4 ounces unsweetened cranberry juice (such as R.W. Knudsen) with 4 ounces of water. Drink once per day at bedtime. You may also have additional servings during the day using 2 ounces of the juice. This juice is very tart, so we highly recommend adding stevia or another non-caloric natural sweetener.

For a tasty mocktail option, combine 4 ounces of cranberry juice with 4 to 8 ounces of sparkling water over ice and add stevia sweetener to taste (see page 235). It becomes a delicious drink you can enjoy regularly.

3. Fiber Supplements

Don't miss our "Scoop on Poop" discussion later in this chapter to better understand why having a healthy bowel movement (or better yet, two or three) each day is essential to health. When you are adding the cleansing component to your Elimination Phase, this becomes even more important because your body needs to rid itself of the toxins being released. One of those routes is through your digestive tract.

We recommend several types of fibers and encourage you to test them before committing to the full dosage recommended on the label. Every woman's body is unique and will therefore respond differently to various fibers. Some women do great with ground flax or chia but get extremely constipated with psyllium. Others love psyllium and report great BMs.

It's best to start slowly. We suggest seeing how you respond to a certain fiber by cutting the recommended dose in half or less. Take only one dose the first day, and then slowly increase your daily dose to the manufacturer's recommendation.

If you get bound up or experience cramps, bloating, or other symptoms with a low dose, switch to a different source of fiber. If your system doesn't do well with one type of fiber, it will often be fine with a different source. A fiber combination with several types of fiber (such as flax, chia, acacia, and apple pectin) in one formula is very effective. As with single-ingredient fiber sources, start slowly and gradually increase.

Take a supplement every night before bed. You may opt for capsules or powder form. Always drink 10 to 12 ounces of water with your supplement, whether you use capsules or powder. Choose one of the fiber supplements from the following list or find a combo source:

- acacia fiber
- apple pectin
- chia seeds
- ground flaxseed
- psyllium husk or powder*

* We do not recommend psyllium for those prone to constipation.

4. Other Supplements

These are other supplements we recommend:

- *Herbal tea with dandelion root:* This tea helps move toxins through your bile/digestive tract. A good brand is Traditional Medicinals EveryDay Detox.
- *Magnesium oxide:* A natural laxative, magnesium also helps regulate blood-sugar levels, facilitates bone and teeth formation, reduces muscle cramps, and promotes relaxation and sleep. Take 200 to 400 milligrams before bedtime with water. This will enhance elimination. As mentioned, the goal is to have bowel movements two to three times per day.
- *Multivitamins:* Choose one that contains B vitamins and key minerals such as selenium and zinc. This supplement helps boost the enzymatic reactions for detoxification.
- *Smooth Move tea:* This herbal natural laxative tea works well for most people experiencing minor constipation. Start with one 8-ounce cup, lightly brewed.
- *Vitamin C:* Additional vitamin C helps with clearing the blood of toxins. Ideal dose is 2,000 to 3,000 milligrams per day.

Note: Many of the supplements and items needed for the gentle cleansing component may be available at your local grocery or health-food store. For those you cannot find locally, we've included a list of our favorite brands with direct online links at EatLiveThriveDiet.com. This website is available as a resource and includes our downloadable worksheets and other bonus content.

5. Body Brushing

This is a health practice that stimulates the lymphatic system to eliminate cellular waste. It increases circulation, improves kidney function, relieves stress, sheds dead skin cells, and can help reduce the appearance of cellulite. Use a dry natural brush designed for this purpose.

Here are some pointers:

- Start at the feet and brush the bottoms and then up the legs in long, smooth strokes.
- Brush each section of skin approximately ten times.
- For proper lymph flow, brush toward the heart/chest area, where the lymph system drains.
- Repeat the same process with the arms, starting with the palms.
- On the stomach and armpits, brush in a circular clockwise motion.
- If you have help, repeat the process on your back.

Activities to Enhance Detoxification

The following activities increase circulation and stimulate the excretion of toxins through the lymphatic system. Although we will discuss only two of them in more depth here, we encourage you to use as many of these as possible:

- body brushing (as mentioned above)
- box breathing
- chewing well and eating slowly
- daily light exercise
- deep breathing
- drinking lots of water
- Epsom-salt bath (1–2 cups)
- massage
- sauna

Box Breathing

This a technique many find very simple and effective. Here's how you do it:

- Breathe in and out of your nose only.
- Be mindful to do deep belly breathing rather than chest breathing.

- Inhale deeply for over four seconds.
- Hold the air for four seconds.
- Exhale slowly for four seconds.
- Repeat this cycle for one to two minutes two to three times per day or when stressed or fatigued.

Combine a brief time of prayer with your box breathing to bring a whole new level of calm.

Deep Breathing

As a former labor-and-delivery nurse and childbirth educator, Danna has seen firsthand the power of deep breathing to relax women in labor. But deep breathing benefits go far beyond the labor room.

Danna has personally used the techniques we'll share here as the last thing she does at night while falling asleep and the first thing she does in the morning upon waking. It's a great way to start the day and a wonderful tool for dealing with stress, improving your health, stimulating your lymphatic system to release toxins, and facilitating oxygenation of your entire body.

Another amazing benefit of proper breathing is the fact that it positively stimulates the vagus nerve, which has been called the captain of the inner nerve center. This crucial cranial nerve travels throughout the body (*vagus* means "wanderer") and is involved in a vast range of essential functions, communicating nerve impulses to every organ in the body. It heads up an important part of the involuntary (parasympathetic) nervous system, which controls heart rate, digestion, breathing, anxiety, depression, and more.

Many things, such as gastric distress, can burden the vagus nerve, with hiatal hernias being very frequent irritants. Poor posture, excess alcohol, stress, fatigue, and anxiety can also inflame the nerve and disrupt its proper function.

If you want to calm your nerves, improve your mood, and enhance cardiac and digestive function, take a deep breath. Literally. By doing intentional abdominal breathing and holding your breath for four to eight counts, you can stimulate the vagus nerve to reset and work more efficiently. It's simple and it's free.

Cleansing Symptoms During the Elimination Phase

Our bodies have their own natural cleansing and detoxification systems. Wow, our own very complex Environmental Protection Agencies! They include our kidneys, livers, and lymphatic, respiratory, and digestive systems.

Whenever you make a healthy change to your diet and lifestyle, as done in the Elimination Phase, your body will respond by releasing increased levels of toxins (especially in fat cells) at a more rapid rate. As you give your body a break from unhealthy foods and begin to drink more water and engage in other healthy practices such as exercise and body brushing, it has more capacity to process and excrete stored toxins.

During the cleansing process, you may initially experience symptoms. We call this a detox crisis, but it's a good crisis because it results in greater health and vitality. The symptoms vary from person to person and can manifest at different times, and many women sail through without any. Common symptoms include headaches, body aches, flu-like symptoms, mental fogginess, constipation or loose stool, gas and bloating, body odor, skin breakouts, light-headedness, congestion, fatigue, and mood swings. The good news is, these symptoms are typically short lived, anywhere from a few hours to one to two days.

> I was amazed at the results of eliminating sugar from my diet. The energy and mental clarity the detox brought has encouraged me to change my eating lifestyle. I have added the cleansing drink as a regular part of my diet, as it reduces cravings and hunger.
>
> —Sheila

Some years ago, Robyn was doing a cleanse and showed up to help a friend pack for a move. Robyn suddenly lost all her energy, and her nose and head got congested. She thought for sure she was coming down with the flu. She drove home and went to bed at 6 p.m., and the next morning she woke up feeling amazing and refreshed, as if nothing had happened. It had been a cleansing crisis.

There are several ways you can lessen cleansing symptoms:

- Drink more water, because it will dilute the toxins being released and help flush them out.
- Take an Epsom-salt bath. The skin is one of the largest organs of the body, and the salt helps draw toxins out of the body. It also eases stress and supports good sleep.
- Drink a small amount of a caffeinated drink. Headaches often occur if you are a regular coffee drinker and have eliminated it cold turkey. If you feel that your headache is from caffeine withdrawal, a small amount of caffeine (such as a quarter cup) will help the headache subside. Continue to eliminate caffeine if possible for Level 3. If you cannot overcome headaches, it may take a longer weaning process to be caffeine free. It is worth discovering how your body can function without it!
- Use magnesium oxide to promote elimination of toxins through bowel movements.
- Try to get extra sleep by going to bed earlier or taking short naps to give your body extra rest to process toxins.

- Stimulate the lymphatic system with dry-skin brushing for more efficient processing of toxins.
- Do deep breathing—it is relaxing and stimulates the lymphatic system.

Maximize Your Elimination Phase

The Importance of Excellent Hydration

Water. Water. Water. We cannot overstate how important excellent hydration is, not only as you begin your Elimination Phase but, quite frankly, always! If you are including the cleansing components during elimination, your body will release toxins more rapidly. Therefore, water is even more essential for flushing them from your body.

Feeling tired or hungry or experiencing headaches can be signs that you need more water. We recommend 64 to 96 ounces of clear noncaffeinated liquids per day.

Evaluating Your Eating Cycle

As we've already discussed, keeping your eating window to twelve or fewer hours per day is very helpful in promoting and maintaining weight loss. Start by considering a twelve-hour fasting period that works for you, such as 8 p.m. to 8 a.m. If you want to realize the added benefits of longer fasting periods, we encourage you to work up to sixteen-hour fasting two to three times per week.

Review the cautions and signs of potential adrenal fatigue noted in chapters 5 and 6 to ensure that the longer fasts are beneficial for you. If you are under excessive stress (physical, mental, or emotional), it is best to keep your fasting window to no more than twelve hours.

Activate Your Body with Activity

Movement and deep breathing stimulate your lymphatic system to pump the sludge of toxins from your body. We can get both by engaging in light exercise.

If your workouts tend to be high intensity or cardio heavy, we recommend that you tone them down a bit if you are on Level 2 or Level 3, as the higher level of detoxification can be taxing to the body when coupled with aggressive exercise. A moderate walk or light workout should be fine no matter what level you choose. We'll discuss the importance of exercise in your health and weight-loss efforts exclusively in chapter 12.

Benefits of Bone Broth

Bone broth is a great addition to your diet, especially during the Elimination Phase. It is abundant in minerals that support the immune system. Bone broth contains amino acids such as glutamine, glycine, and proline that help repair and protect your muscles, joints, and gut. It also aids in the body's natural detoxification process.

The collagen in bone broth helps repair your gut lining, decreases intestinal inflammation, and benefits the skin and joints. It can even help reduce the appearance of cellulite. (Talk about turning back the clock!) Seasoned with sea salt and herbs, bone broth tastes delicious and is perfect for all soup recipes. Unseasoned, it can be added to a smoothie. (See Roasted Chicken Bone Broth recipe on page 223.)

The Scoop on Poop

Let's get personal. There's another kind of elimination to discuss in this phase of the diet: your bowel movements, specifically their quality and frequency. This is important, so don't shy away from this subject!

If you've ever been constipated, you know how uncomfortable and perhaps downright painful it can be. But some of you don't even know you have a problem. As we age, more of us deal with this issue because digestion and elimination slow down. You may have a very sluggish digestive system and without proper "evacuation," your body cannot function ideally.

Whenever we have a question about this fascinating topic (it's fascinating to *us*), we consult Dr. Victoria Bowmann for all the scoop on poop! With a PhD in homeopathy and natural medicine as well as a doctorate in homeopathic medicine, Dr. Bowmann is a pioneer in probiotic research and the benefits of detoxification.

She tells us that the time it takes for food to move from entry to exit is called *transit time.* If that time is too fast, you end up with diarrhea and your body can't absorb all the nutrients in your foods. If the time is too slow, you get constipated and the poop hanging out in your intestines starts to putrefy, increasing your risk of becoming predisposed to disease and illness. Dr. Bowmann says that a seventeen- to twenty-four-hour transit time is ideal.[2] That means that the dinner you ate last night should be eliminated before you eat dinner tonight.

How to Determine Your Transit Time

You can take a corn or red-beet test. If you are not sensitive to corn, eat a quarter cup of organic corn. If you are, then eat some baked red beets.

After you eat the corn or the beets, check your watch. Then wait for the food to appear at the other end. The corn will be obvious, and the beets will turn your poop a deep reddish-purple color. How fun!

Now look at your watch again. How many hours has it been since you swallowed the corn or beets? That's your transit time.

Did We Mention Water?

One of the most common reasons for constipation is not drinking enough water. Dr. Bowmann suggests drinking a *minimum* of half your body weight in ounces of water. (If you weigh 150 pounds, drink at least 75 ounces per day.) Increase that if you are in an extremely hot or dry climate or if you are exercising or doing more intense activity.

Proper hydration is essential for all our bodily systems to perform well, and when the body needs to ration water, it shifts to more immediate needs than keeping our bowels hydrated. As some of you know, passing dehydrated poop can be like a labor-and-delivery experience.

The Fiber Factor

Dietary fiber is another important factor. Mature women need about 25 or more grams of fiber daily. In people groups known for eating lots of plant foods, fiber intake is often 50 to 60 grams per day.

> I am now down forty-two total pounds and lots more inches. It has made a big difference in how I feel and my confidence, and I have been able to keep the weight off so far.
>
> —LaCretia

There are two types of fiber: soluble and insoluble. Think of soluble fiber as a sponge. It helps your stool maintain more water, making it softer and easier to pass through your intestines. In contrast, insoluble fiber is more like a scrub brush and bulking agent. It helps ensure that your intestines don't have a lot of stool residue that can get stuck in little pockets and begin to rot. The bulk it adds also pushes your waste more quickly through the intestines and colon.

Eating two to three servings of fruit and five to seven servings of veggies and other fiber-rich foods every day is the best solution.

However, many of us fall short of that goal. Therefore, a fiber supplement can fill in the gap and keep us regular.

We already shared our recommendations for various fiber supplements during the Level 3 discussion. We highly encourage those of you with elimination issues to consider adding supplements to your diet even if you are starting with Level 1 or 2. Dr. Bowmann has seen great improvement in her clients' overall health when they improve their elimination. Poop on!

Shopping List

FRUITS	VEGETABLES	BEVERAGES	NATURAL SWEETENERS
apples	acorn squash	almond milk (unsweetened)	lo han
apricots	artichokes	coconut milk (unsweetened)	monk fruit extract
avocados	asparagus	cranberry juice (unsweetened)	pure maple syrup
bananas	beets	green tea	raw honey
berries	bell peppers	herbal tea	stevia
grapefruit	bok choy	sparkling water	
grapes	broccoli		**SUPPLEMENTS**
kiwis	brussels sprouts	**OTHER**	choice of fiber supplement
lemons	cabbage	cinnamon	herbal tea w/ dandelion root
limes	carrots	cocoa powder	Lovidia appetite control
mangoes	cauliflower	coconut aminos	magnesium oxide 200–400mg
melons	celery	coconut flour	multivitamin w/ B vitamins
nectarines/peaches	eggplant	raw apple cider vinegar	vitamin C
oranges	garlic	shredded coconut	whey protein powder
papayas	green beans	sunflower seed butter	
pears	herbs	tapioca flour	**FATS**
pineapples	jicama		avocado oil
plums	kale		extra-virgin coconut oil
pomegranates	lettuce (all types)		extra-virgin olive oil
tomatoes	mushrooms		full-fat coconut milk
	parsnips/turnips		ghee (clarified butter)
PROTEINS	pea pods		
beef	peas		
chicken	pumpkin		
eggs	scallions		
fish	shallots		
turkey	spinach		
	sweet potatoes/yams		

Plan for Success

With a bit of planning and the right foods on hand, this diet can be amazingly easy! On the following page, we've included a shopping list of approved foods to help you when you go to the grocery store.

We also recommend that you take the time to review the recipes in chapter 15 and then work them into your menu and snack plan. Doing this will make a huge difference in the quality of your experience, because these recipes can satisfy many of the cravings you may have for some of the foods you've eliminated.

Some of our favorites to help satisfy carb and sweet cravings are Snickerdoodle Muffins (page 192), Dark Chocolate Truffles (page 231), Sun Cookies (page 231), and Lemon Poppy Seed Muffins (page 193).

Healthy Eating Strategies

Here are some suggestions for eating healthily:

- Include protein, fat, and fiber at every meal to promote blood-sugar stability, reduce cravings, and maintain high energy.
- Spread out your carbohydrate intake of fruits and high-glycemic veggies (such as bananas, yams, and sweet potatoes) to one serving every three to four hours to avoid swings in blood sugar. Be sure to limit fruits to three servings per day. We recommend you eat berries for the third serving because they are lower in fructose and carbohydrates.
- A healthy carb boundary to promote blood-sugar stability and reduce insulin resistance is to *never eat more than 30 grams of carbohydrate within a three-hour period.* As an example, a large banana is about 30 grams. An average slice of wheat bread is about 15 grams. A half cup of cooked brown rice is about 21 grams.
- For lunch, choose from any of our recipes or create your own salad or soup with lots of veggies and lean protein. Remember to use sugar-free or homemade salad dressings. Dinner leftovers are a great choice for lunch. You may want to double your dinner recipes for this purpose.
- For snacks, choose from fresh veggies with a healthy salad dressing, berries, bone broth, and muffins. Protein snacks are also excellent because they keep energy high. Hard-boiled eggs or leftover meat or poultry is an excellent snack. We like to roll up a slice of avocado in a slice of turkey.
- For dinner, choose any of the entrée recipes or your own recipes that fit into the food guidelines. For simplicity, choose one of the whey-protein smoothies for a meal on occasion.

Eating Out

Eating out can be a challenge, so we've included a section on this subject (see chapter 11). We give you strategies for staying on track at a wide variety of restaurants. We also share some of our favorite healthy packaged foods.

The Daily Checklist

This checklist is an important tool during the Elimination Phase. Studies show that greater success comes with keeping a daily record of any progress. You can download the checklist at EatLive ThriveDiet.com. If you notice check boxes for actions that you are not incorporating into your diet, simply skip them. We recommend that you take your measurements and weigh on the first day of the Elimination Phase and record these numbers. Weigh at least once per week and record new measurements once a month. We've created a worksheet for this purpose, which can be found at EatLiveThriveDiet.com.

Elimination Phase
Daily Checklist

10 glasses (80 ounces) of water: ☐ ☐ ☐ ☐ ☐ ☐ ☐ ☐ ☐ ☐

☐ ☐ ☐ **Cleansing drink** (5–10 minutes before each meal)

☐ ☐ ☐ **Daily exercise** (at least three 5-minute sessions)   **Total:** _____

☐ **Multivitamin** ☐ **Vitamin C**

☐ **Cranberry drink** (anytime after dinner)

☐ **Fiber supplement** (before bedtime)

☐ **Magnesium oxide** (bedtime)

☐ **12–16 hour fast** (Ideal: 6 p.m. to 8 a.m. or later)   **Total fasting hours:** _____

Rate How You Feel:
In comparison to how you felt on your previous daily diet, please rate these areas one or more times each day. Rate from -5 to +5 with "0" being your norm. Use minus 1–5 if you feel worse and plus 1–5 if you feel better.

My energy level: _____   My sleep: _____   My mental clarity: _____

My digestion: _____   My cravings: _____   My aches and pains: _____

Download a blank version of this worksheet at EatLiveThriveDiet.com.

Move from "E" Phase to "D" Phase

To lock in your changes from the Elimination Phase and continue losing weight if desired, commit to doing the Discovery Phase immediately and do your best to test as many foods as possible. Once that is complete, you'll be ready to create your own personalized eating plan as you enter the Lifestyle Phase. You may choose to go through this process several times as you discover how each level of the diet takes you closer and closer to your goal. We'll discuss this more in chapter 9.

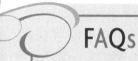

FAQs

Q: What results can I expect in the Elimination Phase?

A: Although individual results vary, improvements are often seen in energy, digestion, concentration, and mental clarity. As for weight loss, most women notice a significant drop on the scale in the first week of elimination because they are no longer eating grains and sugary foods, which tend to hold lots of water. They are also naturally reducing their overall caloric intake because of the elimination of these foods.

Measuring the full scope of your success by the scale is unhealthy, though. It is important to know that slow, steady fat burning is better than losing weight too quickly. Many studies have verified that the female body goes into protection mode and slows down fat burning when a diet produces more than one to two pounds of weight loss per week. For those close to ideal weight, two pounds per week will likely create a similar response.

Choose to evaluate your progress by how your clothes are fitting and how you feel more than by what the scale is saying. Weight loss (if desired) should continue during the Discovery Phase, where you'll realize which foods are causing you weight gain and other health issues. Some of these discoveries can change your life in very positive ways.

Q: There is no mention of calorie or carbohydrate counting or restriction in the Elimination Phase. Do calories count, and is it possible to eat too much of all the "good foods" on the approved list?

A: While calories and carbs certainly do count, it is not important to monitor them when following the Elimination Phase. With the elimination of the troublesome foods—especially sugar and grains—most women naturally reduce their calories.

Also, the diet is lower in carbohydrates (which in many women trigger a negative insulin response), and therefore the calories eaten are burned more efficiently than a diet high in processed foods.

We do caution you, though, to have only one tablespoon of honey or pure maple syrup per day and no more than three servings of fruit. Although you *could* overeat and may even feel as if you're eating more, you are eating the right foods and will soon discover how big of a difference that can make!

Q: If I do choose to monitor calories as well as eliminate foods, how do I know how many calories to eat to lose weight?
A: Except under a doctor's supervision, you should *not* eat less than your basal metabolic rate (BMR) for more than a week or two because you risk slowing your metabolism as your body responds to what it senses to be pending starvation.

You can add two or three days of a 16/8 fasting-and-eating schedule without the risk of lowering your metabolic rate. Your age, weight, height, sex, and muscle mass all affect your BMR. You can get a fairly accurate guesstimate of yours by using the BMR calculator on various websites. Here are two options:

- www.bmi-calculator.net/bmr-calculator
- www.caloriecounter.io/calculators/daily-calories-calculator.html

Q: You mention high- and low-glycemic foods in several places. Which are the high-glycemic foods, and how many can I eat?
A: Some carbohydrate-containing foods cause blood-sugar levels to rise rapidly (high glycemic), while others have a more gradual effect (low glycemic). This is primarily related to the fiber, starch, and natural sugar levels of the food.

The range for high-glycemic foods is 70 and above on the glycemic index (GI). Moderate GI ranges from 56 to 69, and low range is 55 and below.[3] High-glycemic foods (such as bread, pasta, and potatoes) should be eaten in moderation and are metabolized best if combined with protein and fiber.

During the Elimination Phase, you will naturally reduce moderate- and high-glycemic foods. For the Discovery and Lifestyle Phases, we will give you specific guidelines so you can continue to lose weight or maintain the weight loss you have already achieved.

Q: You say that many women are insulin resistant. If I'm not, do I need to reduce moderate- and high-glycemic carbohydrates?

(continued on the next page)

A: The simple answer is yes! If you need to lose excess body fat, chances are that these types of carbohydrates (to include sugar) are the major contributing factors whether you are insulin resistant or not. We've witnessed countless women finally realize weight-loss breakthrough with attention to this issue.

Q: Why are you restricting all grains for each of the three levels of this phase?
A: There are two key reasons we eliminate all grains during the first phase of the diet. First, many women have sensitivities beyond gluten, and they can easily discover these through elimination followed by testing. Second, a large population of women who struggle to lose weight—especially around their middles—have some degree of insulin resistance, which is influenced greatly by the amount or type of carbohydrates they eat.

Not only are most women eating way too many high-glycemic carbs (such as grains), they are also eating them in highly processed forms, such as in crackers, breads, pasta, cookies, and the like. When women remove these completely for fourteen days, they are blown away by how quickly they lose excess water weight, burn fat, and begin to feel better. Their bodies are responding to not only the significant downward shift in both calories and carbohydrates but also a significant decrease in preservatives and additives found in so many of our processed foods.

Patti Milligan estimates that many women eat 300 to 350 grams of carbohydrate each day. If you do the math (at 4 calories per gram), that equals 1,200 to 1,400 calories of carbs! It is likely that most of those calories are not coming from fruits and veggies.

In contrast, during the Elimination Phase, women eat about 80 to 120 grams of carbohydrate, and those will come mostly from the two fruit servings and many vegetable sources. Once you transition to the Discovery and then Lifestyle Phases, your carbohydrate intake can increase a bit. However, to stay lean and healthy, most women will do best if they stay under 200 grams per day and make sure at least half of those are plant based rather than from grains and sugars. We'll discuss this more in chapter 9.

Q: How much water should I drink, and do other liquids count toward that?
A: Ideally, drink 4 to 6 ounces of water for every hour you're awake and more if you are working out or in a hot climate. This should add up to 64 to 96 ounces per day. Herbal tea, other noncaffeinated beverages, and your detox drink count as well. The more water you drink, the easier it is for your body to release the fat.

Q: Is it okay to exercise as usual during Level 3?

A: Keeping naturally active during all levels of the diet is important. Level 3 is unique because your body is releasing more toxins than usual. This increases the workload of many of your organs. High-intensity exercise also produces metabolic waste, so for the fourteen days of Level 3 elimination, walk and do moderate toning exercises only.

Q: Should I still take my prescription medications while in the Elimination Phase?
A: Yes, keep taking your medications, and it's always wise to keep your primary health practitioner apprised of any dietary or lifestyle changes you are making. If you have hormonal issues (for example, diabetes or thyroid dysfunction), a significant change in your diet and weight could alter your dosage requirements.

Q: Should I still take all my current supplements during the Elimination Phase?
A: Yes, you may continue taking them. If you are practicing the ELT Eating Cycle, most supplements are best taken with food for best absorption and to avoid an upset stomach.

Q: Why is the cleansing component important?
A: Detoxification is a natural and continuous process in the body. However, because of today's modern diet, enormous exposure to chemicals (in our food and environment), and the increase in chronic degenerative diseases, a more intentional detoxification is needed for optimal health and metabolism.

Experts agree that all health essentially begins in the gut and is related to the quality of your digestion, absorption, and elimination. The gentle detox/cleansing component of the Elimination Phase allows your body to take a break from many foods, additives, and other compounds that diminish your health and vitality because of a buildup of toxic waste. The goal is to give your digestion a lighter load by taking in only the purest foods that are nutrient dense, plus special drinks and supplements.

Q: Who should not participate in the cleansing component of the program?
A: Pregnant or lactating women should not participate in the cleansing element of the program. If you have a diagnosed kidney or liver disease, heart disease, inflammatory bowel disease, cancer, or any other health concern, you should check with your health-care practitioner.

Q: Are there any potential negative side effects of the cleansing component?
A: As previously mentioned, some people may experience headaches, mental fogginess, unexpected changes in bowel habits, or fatigue during detoxification. One of the primary symptoms is

(continued on the next page)

headaches due to caffeine or sugar withdrawal. These symptoms usually diminish within a few days. If you do experience them, follow the suggestions described earlier to lessen them. And if they do come, say, *Hooray, my body is releasing garbage and I'm getting clean!*

Q: Is it okay to drink the cranberry drink during Level 1 or 2? What are the benefits?
A: Yes, we encourage you to drink this refreshing drink because of its many benefits: blood-sugar stabilization, emulsification of stubborn fat, reduction of water retention, and decrease of systemic inflammation. Think of it as a plunger that activates your lymphatic sewer system to rid itself of waste. (Now, that's a word picture!)

Q: How can I stay on course in Phase 1 or Phase 2 if I frequently eat out at restaurants?
A: We've got you covered! In chapter 11, we give you lots of tips for how to order in various types of restaurants no matter what phase you are in.

Q: Thinking ahead, what should I eat after I complete the Discovery Phase?
A: In chapter 9, which discusses the Lifestyle Phase, we've created two approaches to help you create a customized eating plan based on your Discovery Phase results. You'll choose the foods you may want (or need) to eliminate completely and those you will eat only occasionally because your body responds with negative symptoms. You'll also be given ideas on how to allow yourself some fun foods: those that have little or no nutritional value but do make your life more enjoyable.

In the process of developing your eating plan, we encourage you to repeat Phase 1 (Elimination) for three to seven days if you find yourself veering off course.

Q: Will I still succeed if I don't use the recipes provided?
A: Yes, if you choose to eat the foods in the guidelines along with avoiding the foods on the elimination list. The recipes simply give you some healthy ways to add a tasty variety to your meals and snacks. Many provide a healthy carb-like alternative that can make your diet experience more enjoyable.

Q: What if I mess up? Do I lose all the benefits?
A: Don't stress out about a minor slipup here and there. Just move on and get back on the program as quickly as possible. If you do have a day that is completely off track, consider adding an extra day to your initial week of elimination. Don't quit—just make a fresh start at your next meal!

Elimination Phase
Success Steps at a Glance

- Review the three levels and choose where you'll begin.
- Customize the levels to work for you. For example, choose to eliminate all Level 2 foods and add some of the cleansing components from Level 3. Or choose Level 1 but also eliminate some of the unhealthy foods, such as vegetable oils, shellfish, cold cuts, and cured meats.
- Decide what day you will begin. Tip: It does *not* need to be a Monday.
- For constipation, no matter what Elimination Phase level you choose, add a magnesium supplement each night to improve your transit time.
- Drink 80 to 90 ounces of water daily. Track your water by using a specific-sized container or water bottle.
- Drink the cranberry drink daily regardless of what Elimination Phase level you choose.
- Precook meals on the weekend and refrigerate them to save time during the week.
- Make double recipes of muffins, pancakes, salmon or tuna patties, and so on, and freeze them for convenience.
- Make one of our healthy and tasty salad dressings at the beginning of the week and store it in a jar. When you're going out to eat, take a small container of the dressing with you.
- Be prepared! Carry an apple, hard-boiled egg, or muffin from the recipe list with you so that you always have an option should you find yourself very hungry or if a meal is delayed.
- Create healthy self-talk statements and repeat them to yourself daily (see chapter 4).
- Practice the Eat, Live, Thrive Eating Cycle (short-term fasting).
- Use your daily checklist worksheets, which can be downloaded at EatLive ThriveDiet.com.
- If you start with Level 1, consider notching up to Level 2 or 3 for days 8 through 14.

My food discovery was powerful. First, I learned that sugar is not in control of my life. When I eliminated it, even after just one week, I stopped craving it. I had believed the lie that I would always be addicted to it. I also learned that my body cannot tolerate any dairy. God gave us some amazing foods to eat that are good for our bodies, and when we eliminate the other stuff, he gives us great ideas for enjoying his beautiful food!

—EMMA K.

Transitioning from the Elimination Phase to the Discovery Phase is almost as important as the diet itself. It is at this point that you can unravel the mystery of which foods are holding you back from weight loss and optimal health.

During this stage of the process, you will be adding back only one food at a time. If you don't have a negative response to eggs, dairy, nuts, or legumes, you can leave them in your diet once they've been tested.

However, be mindful that you are very likely adding extra calories or carbohydrates, and this can slow your weight-loss efforts if you are not paying attention. We give you specific recommendations on how much of these foods you should eat in the Lifestyle Phase (see chapter 9). You may want to pop over there to review them as you work through your Discovery Phase.

Because most women who struggle with their weight tend to eat too many grains and too much sugar, especially in the form of processed foods, we take a more conservative approach to testing these foods. You'll notice in the discussion that follows that we ask you to test one grain at a time and then keep that food out of your diet (even if you did not have negative symptoms) until you've tested all grains. This is to help you avoid surpassing your personal carbohydrate and calorie threshold, which we'll discuss more in the next chapter.

At the end of this chapter, we provide a quick "Success Steps at a Glance" synopsis to help you review and decide on the strategies you believe will support you best. We will also share some alternative ways to test various food in the future should you not complete a full test the first time through.

Before we discuss how you will discover your food culprits, it's helpful to reflect on the benefits you experienced from your Elimination Phase. Record your observations here.

My Elimination Phase Results

Weight lost: _____

Inches lost: _____

Digestion: _____

Energy: _____

Mental clarity: _____

Sinus congestion: _____

Cravings: _____

Sleep: _____

Mood: _____

Skin: _____

Aches and pains: _____

Stress or difficulty going through elimination: _____

_____

_____

Download a blank version of this worksheet at EatLiveThriveDiet.com.

Maintaining the Benefits

Look at your answers. If you want to maintain the benefits you've realized from the Elimination Phase, commit to following the Discovery Phase as completely as you can over the next few weeks or more if needed.

This is where you'll potentially unlock the mystery of why you've had difficulty losing weight or have struggled with various symptoms.

Welcoming Back Caffeine and White Potatoes

You can now return to coffee or caffeinated tea if you like. Limit them to no more than two cups per day during the Discovery Phase. If you use milk or cream, be sure you test dairy first. By now we hope you've found a much healthier alternative for sweetening your beverages.

Additionally, you can add white potatoes back into your diet immediately. Limit them to a half cup three times per week. If you love chips, you can enjoy ten to fourteen chips (an ounce) of a healthy brand, such as Boulder Canyon, cooked in avocado or coconut oil. But be careful!

Vegetable Oils

We recommend the long-term exclusion of unhealthy oils, such as canola, soy, and most vegetable oils, which were eliminated during Levels 2 and 3. Instead, use healthy alternatives such as coconut, avocado, and olive oils.

In chapter 10, we'll provide more information about the danger of these oils and why you can help your body turn back the clock by kicking them to the curb permanently.

Let's Get Testing!

As you have learned, some of the foods you restricted during the Elimination Phase are common culprits that disrupt digestion, deregulate blood sugar, exacerbate cravings, and inhibit weight loss. They can also cause overall inflammation in your body, which can be the root of most disease. It is essential to reintroduce these foods one at a time, taking three days to evaluate how each one affects your body. This is the only way you can be sure which foods are causing the problem.

Identifying Your Food Sensitivities

After a period of elimination, you are often more sensitive to the foods that your body dislikes. Therefore, it should be easier for you to notice how they affect your system. Negative reactions can occur within a few hours of eating a food you are reintroducing. However, you may not notice symptoms until the following day, and on occasion it may take two to three days for symptoms to appear.

Have one serving of the test food twice each day for three days. (We define serving sizes specifically in our discussion of each test food.) Carefully monitor your reactions, and then record them on the daily Discovery Phase worksheets. Are you fatigued, foggy headed, bloated, or congested? Are your cravings returning? Did you gain weight?

Water retention or constipation in response to a problem food may cause a quick shift of one or more pounds on the scale. These are all signs that this food may not be the best for your body. If you experience any negative symptoms, remove that food. Do not test another until those symptoms have abated.

If you don't experience anything negative, you can add a new food to test every fourth day. The Discovery Phase worksheets guide you through the entire process. If there is a food listed that you've already eliminated prior to this diet or one you do not like, move to the next food category.

Food Reentry Order

On the following pages, we'll specifically address each food and give you guidelines and recommendations for adding it back into your diet. It is especially important to leave grains and sugar until last. You will notice that we've not included grains such as barley, millet, buckwheat, or rye because they are not as commonly eaten by most people. However, if you eat them often, you may want to test those as well.

We suggest adding back foods in this order:

1. eggs
2. dairy
3. soy
4. nuts and peanuts*
5. legumes (beans)
6. rice
7. oats
8. quinoa
9. corn
10. wheat
11. sugar

*While peanuts are often thought of as nuts, they are actually legumes.

If there is a food on the testing list that you never eat, then by all means skip it. But if you feel "sure" you are not sensitive to a food you do eat, test it anyway. We've seen many women quite surprised to find that a negative symptom they'd been dealing with was caused by one of their favorite foods.

What About Beer, Wine, and Spirits?

For your Discovery Phase to be most accurate, we highly encourage you to avoid alcoholic beverages until you've tested your eliminated foods.

The body reacts to alcohol as a toxin and channels its energy into expelling it. Therefore, other important metabolic processes are interrupted and fat storage is promoted. And your body is not able to store calories from alcohol, so these calories are always burned first, while calories from food have to wait their turn. Additionally, your body's response to alcohol could be confused with reactions from other foods you are testing and you may reach the wrong conclusions.

If you choose to add alcohol right away, make it the first and only "food" you test for the first three days and limit your intake to no more than two servings per day. Danna readily admits that she would gladly give up all chocolate for life rather than go without a full-bodied red wine with a fabulous dinner. For Robyn, it's chocolate that wins the contest. Choose wisely and indulge in moderation to maintain the health and leanness you desire.

Testing Protocol for Each Food

Test Food #1: Eggs

We list eggs first because we want you to be able to use our yummy recipes that can help satisfy those desires for muffins, cakes, cookies, and so on, without all the grains and high carbs.

Eggs can be one of the most digestible and excellent sources of complete protein for many, but for others they may be troublesome. Some symptoms are obvious, while others are discovered only after an elimination diet has been followed.

> *Common symptoms of sensitivity:* upset stomach, flatulence, "shiny" stool that smells like sulfur, a coating on the tongue, a sensation of tightness or closing in the throat.

Not All Eggs Are Equal

An egg is one of the most economical foods you can buy. We believe that it is worth the expense to buy organic, free-range, or (even better) pasture-raised eggs to ensure you get the highest level of nutrition.

> *Serving size:*
> - 1 egg any way you like or included in a recipe (make sure you ingest a full egg for testing purposes)

Test Food #2: Dairy

Dairy can be troublesome for many people. Some symptoms are obvious, while others are discovered only after an elimination diet has been followed for a week or longer.

> *Common symptoms of sensitivity:* upset stomach, gas, bloating, cramps, constipation, skin rash or dryness, acne, congestion or postnasal drip, eye puffiness, weight gain, joint aches and pains.

Not All Dairy Products Are Equal

Conventional dairy products produced in the US present a variety of concerns for the health-minded person. Within the industry, common issues include genetic manipulation, addition of antibiotics and hormones, and less-than-ideal processing via homogenization and pasteurization. These processes leave the milk void of the healthy bacteria our body needs.

> *Recommendation:* Use organic products. Additionally, raw and/or grass-fed milk, cheese, yogurt, and kefir are ideal. Small amounts of standard processed dairy are fine on occasion, but for foods you eat frequently, invest in the highest quality possible. Goat or sheep dairy is a good choice as well. Keep in mind that you may be okay with hard cheeses but have a sensitivity to foods such as cream, yogurt, and milk.
> *Products we like:*
> - Icelandic Provisions yogurt
> - Organic Pastures raw milk, cream, and cheeses
> - Kerrygold grass-fed cheeses and butter
> - Redwood Hill Farm traditional plain goat kefir

- Lifeway Kefir organic whole milk plain kefir
- Maple Hill Creamery organic plain or Greek yogurt

For yogurt and kefir, watch for hidden sugars and fruit juices, as they can increase calories and negatively affect blood-sugar stability and insulin resistance. Use unsweetened options and add a teaspoon of raw honey, stevia, or another natural sweetener of choice.

Serving size:
- 1 cup milk or yogurt
- ½ cup cottage cheese
- 1 ounce hard cheese

Test Food #3: Soy

Soy foods are very popular, especially among vegetarians and people who are sensitive to dairy. Yet along with wheat and dairy, it is one of the top three offending foods in terms of food sensitivities. Sensitivity symptoms may take up to three days to manifest.

Cautions When It Comes to Soy

Some types of soy are much better than others. Much of the soy produced today is genetically modified and linked to many health problems—the glyphosate used in crop production kills off good bacteria in your gut and can wreak havoc on the digestive system.

Plus, soy contains phytoestrogens and goitrogens. Phytoestrogens act as estrogen in the body. For women, excess estrogen can increase the risk of breast and cervical cancers, polycystic ovary syndrome (PCOS), and other hormone issues. Goitrogens can interfere with thyroid production. This type of soy is usually found in soy protein, soy milk, tofu, and most conventional soy products.

Fermented Soy Foods: organic / non-GMO brands of miso, tempeh, natto, tamari

Unfermented Soy Foods (Not Recommended): soy protein, soy milk, soy yogurt, soy ice cream, soy meat (meatless products), edamame, tofu (hemp alternative at some natural-food markets or online)

Soy is also heavy on anti-nutrients such as phytates and lectins, which deplete minerals and disrupt digestion.

On the other hand, fermented soy products such as natto and tempeh are much easier on the gut because after a long fermentation process, the phytates and other anti-nutrient levels drop dramatically.

Dr. Mark Stengler, a naturopathic medical doctor, says, "The most well-studied soy foods to consume for women who want to consume soy without risk are the fermented soy foods. Research also shows that people with normal thyroid function and normal iodine levels do not seem to be susceptible to thyroid problems from soy consumption of any kind."[1]

> *Common symptoms of sensitivity:* fatigue, food cravings, intestinal upset, headaches, runny nose or congestion, breathing issues, skin reactions, itchy mouth, depression, anxiety, panic attacks, attention and focus disruption.
> *Serving size:*
> - 4 ounces tempeh
> - 1 tablespoon miso
> - ½ cup natto
> - 1 cup soy milk (organic, non-GMO)
> - 1 scoop soy protein (organic, non-GMO)
> - ½ cup shelled edamame (organic, non-GMO)
>
> *Soy drink alternatives:*
> - unsweetened almond milk (our fave is Califia Farms)
> - unsweetened coconut milk

Test Food #4: Nuts and Peanuts

Nut allergies are common. If you are allergic to nuts, you are probably already aware of this and will not choose to test this food. If not, you may not be aware that you have an intolerance or sensitivity to them. Some symptoms are obvious, while others are discovered only after the nuts have been eliminated for a time and then tried again.

> *Common symptoms of sensitivity:* upset stomach, gas, bloating, cramps, skin rash or dryness, congestion, itchy mouth, heartburn, headache, weight gain, joint aches and pains, irritability.

Not All Nuts Are the Same

Peanuts are actually legumes and not in the same category as tree nuts, which include but are not limited to almonds, Brazil nuts, walnuts, pistachios, hazelnuts, cashews, macadamia nuts, pine nuts, chestnuts, and pecans.

Therefore, peanuts should be tested on their own. If you are a huge fan of peanuts or peanut butter, test peanuts first and then follow up with the tree nuts.

More Nutty Facts

Nuts can be a great addition to your diet, especially as a snack in small amounts. They include healthy sources of fat, protein, and carbohydrate. Quality nut butters are great for smoothies and work well in many recipes.

But a little goes a long way. Even though these tasty tidbits are packed full of good nutrition, they are also very concentrated sources of fat and calories. A serving size of a quarter cup of shelled nuts is approximately 200 calories. Two tablespoons of nut butter is about 200 calories.

Always choose high-quality organic peanuts or peanut butter because peanuts are one of the most heavily pesticide-sprayed crops. They are also prone to mold and therefore may also be sprayed with a fungicide.

> *Recommendation:* The best source of peanuts are Valencia ones grown in New Mexico. The dry climate eliminates the mold issue. Avoid nut products with added sugar or ingredients other than salt.
>
> *Products we like:*
> - Justin's Nut Butter
> - Arrowhead Mills Creamy Valencia Peanut Butter
> - Costco's or Trader Joe's Organic Valencia Peanut Butter
> - SunButter Organic Sunflower Butter (a seed alternative to nuts)
>
> *Serving size:*
> - ¼ cup nuts and/or seeds
> - 2 tablespoons nut butter or seed butter

Test Food #5: Legumes (Beans)

Most of us have heard the little tune about beans and tooting . . . and some of us have experienced it as well! Beans' natural sweetness comes from a group of sugars called oligosaccharides. Once these sugars reach the large intestines, they are attacked by resident bacteria and create hydrogen and methane gases. As the gas accumulates, it needs a way of escape. That is when the poor dog often receives the blame!

Everyone's body has a unique ecosystem of gut bacteria. The type of bacteria and enzymes you have in your body will make a difference as to how much gas you create when you eat certain foods (not just beans).

> *Common symptoms of sensitivity:* gas, loose stool, abdominal cramps, bloating, weight gain.
>
> *Recommendation:* Be sure that the beans you test have been properly prepared to minimize the bloating effects. They should be soaked for at least twenty-four hours or simmered at 140°F for three hours, eliminating 30 to 70 percent of the phytic acid. Adding baking soda or ½ teaspoon of vinegar to the water will also help you enjoy them without the uncomfortable aftereffects.
>
> If you are using canned beans, buy organic if possible. We recommend you rinse them because the liquid is hard to digest.
>
> If you determine that your body tolerates legumes well, still limit them to two servings per week because of the phytates they contain.
>
> *Serving size:*
> - ½ cup cooked beans

Test Food #6: Rice

Rice is the first grain you will test. It is easily tolerated by most people. However, women with significant sensitivity to grains in general may have sensitivity to rice as well.

> *Common symptoms of sensitivity:* fatigue or low energy, mental fogginess, gas, bloating, upset stomach, constipation, congestion, joint aches and pains, weight gain.

Not All Rice Is Equal

Brown rice has more fiber and nutritional value than white rice because white rice has had the germ and bran removed. One small benefit of white rice is that it is easier to digest. However, white rice is high on the glycemic index and can produce a negative insulin response.

For those prone to insulin resistance, neither brown nor white versions are good choices on a regular basis. Long-grain rice has a lower glycemic load than short-grain rice. Of all the choices of long-grain rice, basmati seems to have the lowest glycemic load of all. We also recommend buying organic to avoid pesticides and other chemicals. Plus, organic rice has a much lower level of arsenic.

Serving size:
- ½ cup cooked rice

Test Food #7: Oats

Oats, a favorite among many people, have received positive press because of their ability to help reduce serum-cholesterol levels. Generally oats do not create any significant digestive issues. But for some, the phytic acid and the avenin (a protein like gluten in wheat) can cause sensitivity and intolerance. This can exacerbate leaky-gut syndrome in some people.

Common symptoms of sensitivity: mental fogginess, lethargy, upset stomach, gas, bloating, cramps, constipation, congestion or postnasal drip, weight gain, depression.

Oats and Gluten Contamination

Oats do not naturally contain gluten. However, sources in the US are frequently cross-contaminated in the milling process, because the same machines and trucks are used for both oats and wheat. Therefore, look for a gluten-free source of oats.

Product we like: Bob's Red Mill Gluten-Free Oats
Serving size:
- ½ cup cooked oatmeal
- ¼ cup dry oats used in a recipe (such as meat loaf)

Test Food #8: Quinoa

Many people consider quinoa a perfect health food. However, for some this seed (not grain) is not easily digested and causes many of the sensitivity symptoms noted below. The main reason is because it is high in compounds known as saponins. Quinoa has properties very similar to those of wheat even though some people use it as an alternative for gluten grains.

Common symptoms of sensitivity: upset stomach, gas, bloating, cramps, constipation, skin rash or dryness, congestion or postnasal drip, fatigue, low energy, moodiness, depression, headaches, weight gain, joint pain or stiffness.

Recommendation: Quinoa registers 53 on the glycemic index. For those with insulin resistance, this food can convert to fat quite easily. If you choose to eat it, wash it well because its outer coating is responsible for some of its wheat-like properties.
Serving size:

- ½ cup cooked quinoa

Test Food #9: Corn

Corn is difficult to avoid because it is included in many processed foods. Unfortunately, a large percentage of this corn is genetically modified. That is why eating whole foods and staying away from packaged and processed choices help you know exactly what you are eating.

Ingredients that (unexpectedly) contain corn include:

- caramel
- dextrin
- dextrose
- fructose
- high-fructose corn syrup (HFCS)
- malt syrup
- modified food starch
- vinegar

Common symptoms of sensitivity: muscle weakness, joint pain, stomach cramps, bloating, constipation, loose stool, lack of energy, speech problems, headaches, hyperactivity, mood swings, depression, insomnia, fine-motor-skills issues, undigested food in stool.

Non-GMO Versus GMO

Genetically modified corn contains formaldehyde and glyphosate—both toxic. The glyphosate has been linked to liver damage in animals. When given the choice between the two types of corn, animals will always go for the real corn and avoid the GMO. Let's follow the herd on that decision!

Recommendation: If your body tolerates corn, choose non-GMO and organic. Read labels carefully because many foods contain hidden sources of corn. Most corn on the cob is non-GMO, but check with your local grocer to be sure. If a product is truly non-GMO, it should include the logo or words *non-GMO project verified.*

Product we like: Popcornopolis Nearly Naked Popcorn. It is certified non-GMO popcorn made with coconut oil. It is Danna's favorite go-to snack and can be found at Costco and online.

Serving size:

- ½ cup cooked corn or 1 ear of corn
- 10 tortilla chips
- 2 (6-inch) corn tortillas
- 3 cups popped popcorn

Test Food #10: Wheat

Look at "Ancient Grains" (page 100) for a discussion on wheat. When it comes specifically to modern wheat, it is completely different from historic wheat because of the milling processes used and because the seed itself has been genetically modified since the mid-1950s.

Many experts have linked eating processed wheat with impaired weight loss. As we've already mentioned, the conventional processing and packaging of wheat in the US lead us to conclude that it is a food that all women should eat sparingly whether or not they are actually sensitive to wheat and/or gluten. Sensitivity may not manifest in a person until later in life. In fact, most people who have gluten intolerance are never diagnosed.

Common symptoms of sensitivity: bloating, headaches, joint pain or swelling, numbness in extremities, indigestion, gas, constipation, diarrhea, nervousness, mood swings, low energy, fatigue, mental fogginess, changes in skin, rash, sleep disturbances, weight gain. In some cases, people experience weight loss due to poor absorption. However, that is not the kind of weight loss you want!

Recommendation: Substitute coconut or almond flour in recipes. Use tapioca or arrowroot flour for dredging (breading) and thickening sauces. For some, Ezekiel bread (sprouted grain) and traditionally made sourdough bread (fermented for at least seven hours) are more easily digested.

Serving size:

- 1 slice bread or ½ hamburger bun
- ¾ cup cooked noodles
- ½ bagel or English muffin
- 1 medium flour tortilla
- 1 slice pizza crust

Grain-Testing Recommendations

Grains. It's hard not to love the satisfaction of biting into a warm, aromatic slice of freshly baked bread. Or how about the fiesta of flavor you experience when you take your first bite of a freshly made crispy tortilla chip? Sigh.

Grains are comfort foods for many of us, and whether a part of a favorite family recipe or a nibble on the run, they satisfy us in a way many foods do not. Most of us eat way too many unhealthy sources of grains, mostly in the form of processed and packaged breads, cereals, crackers, and desserts. The food pyramid of the nineties instructed us to eat at least six grain servings every day. We now know that not only do these tasty morsels provide us with a lot of excess calories and carbohydrates, but they are also causing other health issues such as inflammation. And many people cannot properly digest some grains due to food sensitivities. With the skyrocketing increase in insulin resistance, obesity, and the risk of diabetes, it makes sense to rewire our perspective about grains. Most women need to put grains at the top of the food pyramid as an occasional indulgence rather than at the bottom as a staple.

That's why we have you remove them all during the Elimination Phase. Doing so gives your body a chance to heal, and your carbohydrate and calorie intake immediately decreases. You see the results. You drop weight. Your cravings diminish. Your energy increases and you feel better overall. But most of us don't want to live without grains forever. Don't worry—we're here to help *you* find *your* answers.

Ancient Grains

We're often asked, "If grains are mentioned in Scripture and have been eaten for thousands of years, how could they not be good for us?" The answer lies in the fact that hundreds of years ago, grains were harvested and prepared differently. Traditional methods of soaking, sprouting, and fermenting were used to make the grains easier to digest and slowed the conversion of carbohydrates into sugars in the body.

With the influx of paleo and keto diets, grains have become vilified. God created grains for food, but we humans have corrupted many of them. Quality grains in their most natural state provide vitamins and minerals not accessible in other foods. Their level of B vitamins is especially important. And although we can certainly supplement, there is no better place to find the best quality of nutrients than within the foods God has created for us.

Processed Wheat

Our expert Patti Milligan believes there is more sensitivity to wheat because of how it is processed and preserved rather than because of the gluten itself. This is also true for many other grains, such as corn, that are often genetically modified. We don't need to throw out all grains permanently; we just need a new plan. The challenge is to find the most healthy sources of grains and discover which ones our bodies handle best. We also want to discover just how many grains we can eat if we want to lose weight or maintain it.

One Grain at a Time

As part of your discovery in this important area, each grain should be tested separately. You will test for not only food sensitivity but also your response to adding this extra carbohydrate load twice each day. Depending on your carbohydrate threshold, this addition may destabilize your blood sugar. The additional calories coupled with the increased glycemic load can begin reversing some of your great results quite quickly. Therefore, control your portion sizes and eat only two servings each day of the specific grain you are testing.

As you move to the next grain, delete the previous grain from your diet—even if you didn't have any negative symptoms—so you're not taking in too many carbohydrates and calories. We'll discuss this in more detail and help you discover your personal carbohydrate threshold in the Lifestyle Phase (see chapter 9).

Test Food #11: Sugar

Sugar is everywhere! It seems impossible to avoid because it's hidden in so many foods, such as cereal, condiments, sauces, salad dressings, marinades, peanut butter, soups, and juice. The list goes on and on. And who doesn't love chocolate or special desserts!

As infants, many of us were nourished by naturally sweet breast milk, and we are instinctively drawn to most foods with natural sweetness, like bananas. God created us with "sweet" taste buds, and he clearly gave us the ability to discern and enjoy sweet foods. But somewhere in years past, we took something natural and good and became a society of sugar junkies.

> I discovered that when I ate wheat products, some of the joints in my fingers became very tender. When I cut the products out, pain gone!
>
> —Mary

The average American consumes approximately sixty-six pounds of added sugar every year, according to the US Department of Agriculture (USDA). Several hundred years ago, the figure was only about four pounds per person.[2]

For some people, sugar affects the reward center in their brains to such an extent that it seems to act like an opioid drug, such as morphine and heroin. For them, this makes sugar almost impossible to resist. Dr. Mark Hyman, director of the Cleveland Clinic Center for Functional Medicine, states, "Sugar is eight times as addictive as cocaine."[3]

By Any Other Name

Sugar has many names, including high-fructose corn syrup, fructose, dextrose, glucose, sucrose, agave, cane juice, brown-rice syrup, and barley malt.

Why Is Sugar Harmful?

Too much sugar promotes disease and inflammation. It is also the preferred nourishment source for cancer cells. It decreases our overall immunity and can lead to many other serious conditions, such as

- arthritis and joint inflammation
- diabetes
- emotional disruption and behavioral problems
- heart disease
- immune disruption

- migraines
- obesity

To Test or Not to Test?

The truth is, none of us needs processed sugar in our diets. We can get plenty of natural sugar through fruits and other sources, such as raw honey and pure maple syrup. Now that you've removed sugar, you've likely noticed that your cravings have diminished and your energy has soared. The best thing you can do is stay on the course you are now without adding sugary treats back in.

If you do decide to test sugar, you want to watch specifically for an immediate spike in hunger and cravings. Watch the scale closely and see what happens. You want to not only be on the lookout for the common sensitivity symptoms noted below but also pay special attention to your sugar threshold. That is the amount of sugar you can eat and still feel in control. When cravings increase, you've moved into the danger zone. You'll notice that the serving sizes we recommend during testing are very small.

> *Common symptoms of sensitivity:* low energy, lethargy, headaches, moodiness, irritability, depression, low self-esteem, lack of creativity, joint aches, weight gain. In addition, fructose has been known to cause digestive upset, cramps, diarrhea, and gas.
>
> *Serving size:*
> - 1 ½ ounces chocolate
> - 4 ounces fruit juice
> - ½ cup ice cream
> - 1 tablespoon strawberry jam
> - 1 cookie (2-inch diameter)
>
> *Sugar Alternatives:*
> - Use natural sweeteners, such as stevia, monk fruit, and lo han.
> - Use limited amounts of organic raw honey or pure maple syrup.
> - Sweeten with small amounts of dates, applesauce, or bananas in some recipes.

Note: If you are fructose sensitive, keep in mind that honey, maple syrup, dates, and fruit contain fructose.

Sweeteners we like:

- pure monk fruit extract
- liquid or powdered stevia
- granulated stevia and monk fruit organic sweetener (packets only)
- liquid lo han drops

Your Discovery Begins Now!

Are you ready to begin testing? We're excited for you to unravel some of the mysteries surrounding your weight and health challenges. Think of this time as a science experiment of sorts and you are the primary subject! We hope you'll unlock the door to lasting change by making some key discoveries as Sandi did.

I now know what foods I should avoid for overall health and weight management, and I've found so many wonderful foods that fuel my body and give me energy. In the past six months, I have lost twenty-five pounds and twenty-eight overall inches. I feel like I've rolled back the clock twenty years! —Sandi (age fifty-seven)

Let us emphasize this one more time: the Discovery Phase is very important, and it is worth doing well. If you mess up, just start fresh the next day by eliminating any foods that you should not have eaten. Wait until any negative symptoms abate, and then begin testing again.

> Most people think oats are really healthy, and they can be. But for others, not so much. When I eat oats, they put me into a two-hour brain fog!
>
> —Robyn

Daily Discovery Worksheets

To learn the most from your Discovery Phase, take the time to complete a daily worksheet for each food tested. It takes only a few moments to complete each day, and the worksheet has some reminder check boxes at the bottom to keep you practicing your new healthy habits. You can find free downloadable worksheets on our website at EatLiveThriveDiet.com. Just register and enjoy the extra resources there to help you on your journey. We've included an example worksheet to help you get started.

Day #: _1_

New Food: _dairy_   **Morning Weight:** _146_

Type Eaten: _organic half-and-half_   Amount: _2 tablespoons_ Time: _8 a.m._

Type Eaten: _grass-fed cheddar_   Amount: _1 ounce_   Time: _3 p.m._

Type Eaten: _low-fat cottage cheese_   Amount: _½ cup_   Time: _6 p.m._

Eliminated Foods I Ate Prematurely:

Type Eaten: _peanuts_   Amount: _¼ cup_   Time: _11 a.m._

Type Eaten: _____   Amount: _____   Time: _____

Physical and Emotional Observations:

Digestion: _A little gassy today!_

Energy: _Same—good_

Mental Clarity: _Okay_

Sinus Congestion: _Just a tad stuffy_

Cravings: _Under control!_

Mood: _Pretty good_

Other: _Will eat less tomorrow and not eat the peanuts and see if gas is gone_

Habits I'm Continuing:

Total Ounces of Water Today: _88_   **ELT Eating Cycle:** _12-hour fast_

[X] Daily Exercise   [X] Deep Breathing   [X] Cleansing Drink

[ ] Body Brushing   [X] Supplements   [X] Cranberry Drink

Download a blank version of this worksheet at EatLiveThriveDiet.com.

Discovery Phase
Success Steps at a Glance

- Test only one new food at a time, and skip any foods you don't eat regularly.
- Eat two portions per day of the food you are testing, being mindful of recommended portions.
- Test a new food every four days unless you notice sensitivity symptoms.
- Stop eating any food that provokes a sensitivity, and do not test another food until symptoms are gone, usually within two or three days.
- Test dairy first if you use milk or cream in your coffee/tea.
- Test as many different foods as possible. If you don't get through all the foods, you can circle back in a month and repeat the Elimination and Discovery Phases and test the foods you missed.
- Continue to use the recipes that you enjoyed during your Elimination Phase to stay satisfied.
- Practice new, beneficial habits and supplements, such as the ELT cleansing drink, the cranberry drink, magnesium, and fiber.
- Use the Discovery Phase daily worksheets, which can be downloaded for free at EatLiveThriveDiet.com.
- Weigh yourself at the beginning of Discovery and then every day or two to see what foods may be negatively affecting your weight.

I don't believe in diets. All I hear is the word *die*! The Eat, Live, Thrive Diet is a sustainable lifestyle in which you eat real food. The gift of food is received and enjoyed as it was intended to be by our Creator.

—DIANA

Woo-hoo! You've made it to the Lifestyle Phase! Whether you completed the full Discovery Phase or just tested a few foods, you've most likely gained some important insights.

Even if you did not discover any specific food sensitivities, you probably realized that you feel better and can lose weight more easily when you greatly reduce grains, sugar, and processed foods. Most of us know that, but until we experience the full benefits, our cravings often override the desire to be leaner and healthier. As we discussed, you can get creative with your Elimination and Discovery Phases. You may prefer doing a seven-day elimination each month followed by a short discovery period in which you'll test only two or three foods. Our goal in this chapter is to help you determine the best way to use the three phases of this program to reach your goals.

Embrace the Journey

Your lifestyle journey is a work in progress. Give yourself time and grace to let it evolve as you take small consistent steps toward lasting change. We hope you will go through the three phases many times over the years ahead as part of that journey.

There will be many tips and strategies to consider in this chapter. We don't want you to feel as though you need to implement everything at once. At the end of this chapter, we provide a quick "Success Steps at a Glance" synopsis to help you review and get started.

Although ideal nutrition is the goal, it's important to be realistic about how much change you can effectively take on all at once. Don't fall into a perfection mind-set in which your attitude is "all or nothing." Many studies show that even improving your nutrition by 10 to 20 percent *consistently* can significantly enhance your health and promote weight loss.

Keep coming back to the basics of this plan and what you've learned. If you do what you can each day to improve your nutrition—not to mention other positive lifestyle habits such as good sleep, regular exercise, and stress management—you will see each small change begin to add up in big ways over time.

We completely understand the challenge. Both of us have had our own obstacles to overcome regarding food and body issues (see our stories in the introduction!). If we can lock in permanent changes, so can you. If you don't give up, you will gain victory.

Creating a Sustainable Lifestyle Eating Plan

Now comes the important part: developing a *sustainable* eating plan that will work for you. We define *sustainable* as something you can do most days and still enjoy your life!

> I'm down twelve pounds! I'm doing best with no dairy, grains, sugar, or corn. I found that I'm allergic to almonds and get a rash on my neck. The pain and inflammation in my hands and knees is gone. My skin has cleared up and my eyes look brighter. I have more energy and the sugar cravings are gone. I just look and feel better. I love this program. It's very doable and easy. Thank you!
>
> —Shelley

That does not mean that you will give yourself permission to eat tons of empty calories; it means you will find the balance between excellent nutrition and just enough fun foods to keep you happy and following your plan steadily.

It is in the daily consistency that we realize our greatest and lasting benefits. As those benefits increase, you will look and feel better. That will become your new motivation rather than the desire for immediate "taste gratification."

Take the time necessary to create and modify your eating plan over the weeks and months ahead until you've landed on something you truly believe you can do regularly. In our personal journeys, our own lifestyle diets have continually evolved as we learn new things about our responses to certain foods and are enlightened about new nutritional science.

For example, I (Danna) can eat almost anything and not gain weight if I keep my calories under control. But I notice that after a few days of eating wheat products, the arthritis in my hands is more painful. I know from research that wheat-based foods can cause inflammation throughout the body, so I have chosen to greatly reduce my consumption.

After enjoying a variety of nuts for many years, I (Robyn) started noticing that some caused bloating. I also tended to overeat them because they did not give me any sense of satiation. So now I often exclude most of them from my diet.

We did not uncover these sensitivities in our first rounds through the Elimination and Discovery Phases. You will likely have similar experiences, and that is why we encourage you to cycle through the three phases throughout the year in creative ways.

Before designing your lifestyle plan, consider these important questions:

- Are you willing to eliminate or drastically reduce the foods that you know are unhealthy or produce unwanted symptoms when you eat them?
- Even if you did not experience any obvious signs of sensitivity, will you consider reducing your intake of high-glycemic carbohydrates from grains and sugars, especially those found in packaged and processed foods?
- What will that reduction be for you? 25 percent? 50? 75? 90? We recommend the 90/10 boundary, allowing yourself grace for 10 percent fun food on occasion as a healthy baseline.
- What is your motivation to change your eating? Is it weight loss? Better health? More energy? Longevity and anti-aging benefits? By keeping your focus on your biggest motivation, you'll increase your ability to succeed.
- Are you willing to work on your inner dialogue in the areas where you struggle so you can rewire your automatic responses with new, healthier messages?

The worksheet on the following page, which can be downloaded from EatLiveThriveDiet.com, allows you to record the foods you plan to eliminate from your diet because of sensitivity or perhaps strong emotional ties that trigger overeating.

Designing Your Lifestyle Diet

Let's take a moment to dig deeper into a few subjects that will help you make decisions so you can sustain the fat-burning and health benefits you've realized thus far. We encourage you to start where you are and make changes to your diet that you can sustain. If you feel as though you're in a constant state of deprivation, you'll probably fall off the wagon.

Our goal is to help you make changes that are doable and find substitutions for unhealthy foods so you never feel deprived.

Lifestyle Phase
My New Food Choices Worksheet

Foods I will remove almost completely:

1. _____ Why? _____

2. _____ Why? _____

3. _____ Why? _____

4. _____ Why? _____

Foods I will eat only occasionally:

1. _____ Why? _____

2. _____ Why? _____

3. _____ Why? _____

4. _____ Why? _____

Foods I will increase in my diet:

1. _____ Why? _____

2. _____ Why? _____

3. _____ Why? _____

4. _____ Why? _____

My weight goal: _____ **My size goal:** _____

My health goals: _____

_____

Download a blank version of this worksheet at EatLiveThriveDiet.com.

Carbohydrates and Calories

We want to circle back to the importance of carbohydrate and calorie levels. They both matter, and you will need to determine how much of each will support your goal of a leaner body.

Perhaps you are wondering why we did not discuss this specifically at the beginning of the diet. That's because we know from vast experience that if you follow the Level 1, 2, or 3 guidelines, you will likely lose weight without counting calories or carbohydrates.

Why You Lost Weight

During the Elimination Phase, you significantly reduced your high-glycemic carbohydrates, such as white potatoes, grains, and all sources of sugar except the one tablespoon of organic raw honey or pure maple syrup per day. You also eliminated fruit juices and limited your fruits to three servings because of the naturally occurring fructose.

These high-glycemic carbs raise your blood sugar quickly and therefore trigger a more profound insulin response. This creates a blood-sugar roller coaster, resulting in increased cravings, decreased energy, and diminished immunity. These foods are also the number one source of excess calories and unhealthy fats. When you remove or greatly decrease the consumption of these foods, it makes a dramatic impact on your health and weight loss rather quickly.

In addition, there may have been some troublesome foods that were inhibiting your weight loss. If the symptoms you noticed during the Discovery Phase were mild, be mindful of any weight gain should you decide to eat them on occasion.

Your Lifestyle Home Base

You may wonder why we are spending time reminding you of how and why you lost weight and felt better during the Elimination Phase. It's because we want you to appreciate the powerful results and realize that Phase 1 can be your home base for resetting and rebooting your eating plan whenever you catch yourself veering off track.

Let's continue looking at why you lost weight:

- Eating only the approved foods reduced your carbohydrates and calories naturally. As mentioned in chapter 7, we estimate that most women eat 80 to 120 grams of carbohydrate per day during the Elimination Phase.
- It's rare to overeat the approved nutrient-dense foods because they keep you full, support blood-sugar stability, and reduce cravings. This usually results in an added benefit of increased energy. When you feel good, your appetite is more naturally under control.

- Unlike grains, sugar, and other high-glycemic foods, the approved foods do not readily convert to stored fat.
- Avoiding sugar and white flour reduces your cravings, which helps you stay on track.
- When nutrition is balanced, the body is better able to release fat.
- The detox/cleansing component helps your body release toxins and become better prepared to break down and release fat.
- Eliminating potentially troublesome foods may have prompted your body to more effectively lose weight.

Fact: All Carbohydrates Are Not Equal

As you discovered, the lower-glycemic veggies can be eaten without limit. Fruits have great nutritional value, but most are higher on the glycemic index than veggies and therefore do need limits.

However, the fiber in the higher-glycemic plant foods (such as carrots, bananas, and apples) slows the release of the carbohydrates into your system and therefore makes these foods better choices than most grains, starches, or processed foods. You will see in our recommendations later in this chapter that we advise decreasing your daily fruit intake to two servings per day because you are reintroducing more starches (which you were not eating during the Elimination and Discovery Phases). However, if you don't add grains or other high-glycemic foods, feel free to add an extra fruit.

Fact: Sugar and White Flour Are the Deadly Duo

The two worst offenders of all the foods you eliminated are sugar and white flour. You knew that. They have almost no nutritional value beyond providing calories for energy.

They decrease your immunity, promote fat storage, and increase insulin resistance. We consider them edible poisons that can slowly kill us if we eat them too often. But we confess that we eat them on occasion!

From Eliminated Foods to Caution Foods

Once you've determined which eliminated foods you can eat without negative symptoms, you'll need to discover how many of those you can add back into your diet and still lose or maintain weight. We'll now refer to these foods as caution foods. These foods are not necessarily bad when eaten occasionally but can become your nemeses if you eat too many too often. Some of the foods increase your carbohydrate load, and others are high in calories. A few are both.

Every woman has her unique carbohydrate and caloric thresholds. That is how much her body can assimilate without having a negative impact on her weight, health, cravings, and energy. As you carefully add these foods (especially grains) into your diet, you'll quickly discover how they affect your weight and how you feel.

Patti Milligan recommends thinking of grains as condiments rather than staples. This helps put the amount you consider eating into a very different perspective.

We recommend not exceeding 150 to 200 grams of total carbohydrates per day during the Lifestyle Phase. Don't worry—you don't have to count if you choose to use our "Keep It Simple" approach, which we'll explain shortly.

Portions Matter

One of your biggest challenges will be adding previously restricted foods in a way that keeps you satisfied without sabotaging your weight loss. Most of us have misconceptions when it comes to serving sizes. Take the time to pull out your measuring cups or small weight scale and become very familiar with what a healthy portion looks like.

Daily portion recommendations are as follows:
- dairy: 1–2 servings (see list on page 116 for portion size)
- fruits: in moderation (2–3 servings) depending on your starch intake
- healthy fats: up to 3 tablespoons per day
- nuts: ¼ cup per day
- proteins: up to 4 servings per day (4–6 ounces)
- starches (grains, corn, potatoes, beans): 2 servings per day maximum
- sugar: 2 tablespoons raw honey or pure maple syrup
- vegetables: unlimited (excluding potatoes and corn)

What About Wheat?

Even if you are not sensitive to wheat, consider adding no more than two servings per week unless you are baking your own foods or buying them from a local bakery that has quality wheat sources not processed in the US. As mentioned in chapter 1, all American conventional wheat is washed with chlorine, and many food manufacturers are adding unhealthy additives and preservatives to their products.

Confession: we *do* indulge on occasion. Robyn may snag a piece of her husband's pizza when they're dining out, and Danna admits she cannot resist the San Francisco–style sourdough bread at her favorite seafood restaurant. But these are exceptions to our everyday lifestyle practices. Admittedly, it has taken us quite a few years to transition to our current lifestyles.

Give yourself grace and make a commitment to ponder what is going on inside your body after you swallow those tasty morsels. That focus has helped us both say no more often than yes, and we feel as if we are nurturing rather than depriving ourselves.

Hazard Food!

Sugar is in a category all its own, far beyond the "caution food" category. It is one of the most disruptive anti-nutrients on the planet and a major causative factor in many diseases. It is well documented that cancer craves sugar and avoiding it is instrumental in prevention and cure.

This is what Ty Bollinger, medical researcher and best-selling author, says:

> Whether you are currently healing from a type of cancer such as breast cancer or prostate cancer, or are simply trying to maintain good dietary principles, I personally recommend that you avoid white sugar, brown sugar, agave, and all artificial sweeteners such as aspartame/AminoSweet, sucralose, and saccharin. If you have a sweet tooth, it's best to stick with 100% organic green stevia, xylitol, raw honey, pure maple syrup, molasses, and coconut sugar.
>
> The bottom line . . . if you want to be and stay healthy, you MUST take control of your sugar intake so that it doesn't take control over you and your health![1]

So How Much Sugar Is Okay?

Many of us need to cut sugar out of our diets completely because it is essentially addictive for us. However, most of us want a little sweet now and then. Of course, one to two tablespoons of organic raw honey or pure maple syrup per day would be ideal. We could all benefit from this level of discipline.

But we will probably cave in to the white stuff on occasion. The thought of never having a conventional sweet treat makes us want it that much more, right? For those in that boat, limit added sugar or sweet treats to a maximum of two sweet treats per week.

Two Strategic Lifestyle Approaches

We've designed two approaches to help you develop a sustainable eating plan. Robyn's preference, the "Keep It Simple" approach, provides specific food groups and servings permitted each day. Danna's preference, the "By the Numbers" approach, allows you to choose the amount and frequency of each food and focus on accountability through monitoring your calorie and carbohydrate intake.

Approach #1: Keep It Simple

If you're a woman who hates details, you might like this plan and the daily diet worksheet we've created, which allows you to log the foods you eat based on the serving recommendations. The foundation of this plan is similar to how you ate during the Elimination Phase; plus it strategically adds the tested foods that your body responded well to. By following the recommendations, you will be naturally controlling your carbohydrate and calorie levels.

Second to sugar, starchy foods are the main culprit causing weight gain in women. Because these foods are higher on the glycemic index, limiting them will keep your diet in balance. Although nuts and dairy are less troublesome, they can add a lot of excess calories if portions are too large or they are eaten too often.

As you begin testing your new lifestyle diet, track your weight, cravings, and energy. If those are changing for the worse, it's time to course correct and lower the number of servings per day of those caution foods. We've included a partial list of caution foods with recommended portion sizes. Of course, if you tested sensitive to any of these foods, it is wise not to eat them on a regular basis.

Starches: 1–2 servings per day

beans: *½ cup, cooked*
bread: *1 slice*
cereal: *see package for serving size*
cooked corn: *½ cup or 1 ear*
corn tortilla: *2 (4"–6" diameter)*
couscous: *½ cup, cooked*
dinner roll: *1*
dried fruit: *¼ cup*
English muffin: *½ muffin*
flour tortilla: *1 (6"–8" diameter)*
french fries: *10 fries*
fruit juice: *4 ounces*
granola bar: *1 bar*
hamburger or hot dog bun: *½ bun*
oats: *½ cup, cooked*
pancakes: *2 (4" diameter)*
pasta and noodles: *¾ cup*
pizza crust: *1 slice*

popcorn: *3 cups, popped*

potato, sweet: *½ baked potato or ½ cup, mashed*

potato, white: *½ baked potato or ½ cup, mashed*

potato chips: *approximately 14 chips*

pretzels: *see package for serving size*

quinoa: *½ cup, cooked*

rice: *½ cup, cooked*

rice cakes: *2 cakes*

tortilla chips: *approximately 10 chips*

Packaged Snack Options: 1 serving per day

Clif Bars: *½ bar (1 starch serving)*

dried fruit: *¼ cup (1 starch serving)*

KIND Nut Bars: *1 bar*

Perfect Bars: *½ bar (1 starch serving)*

plantain chips: *approximately 20 chips (1 starch serving)*

nut butter or seed butter: *2 tablespoons*

nuts: *¼ cup*

Dairy: 1–2 servings per day

cheese: *1 ounce*

cottage cheese: *½ cup*

kefir: *8 ounces*

half-and-half: *6 tablespoons*

plain yogurt: *6 ounces*

sour cream: *6 tablespoons*

Keep It Simple: Worksheet Directions and Guidelines

As you can see from our example on the following page, this worksheet helps you track the daily servings from each key food category.

Vegetables

There are six spaces for vegetables, and we encourage you to use them all—and even more if possible. Vegetables are filling, high-volume foods with tons of nutrients and fiber. Eat them liberally!

My Weight Today: _153_

Vegetables	Amount	Vegetables	Amount
1. zucchini	1 medium	4. broccoli	1 cup
2. mushrooms	¼ cup	5. grape tomatoes	9
3. cabbage	2 cups	6. spaghetti squash	2 cups

Fruits	Amount	Fruits	Amount
1. apple	1 medium	2. blueberries	½ cup

Proteins	Amount	Proteins	Amount
1. egg	1	3. tuna	6 ounces
2. turkey sausage	3 links	4. chicken	approx. 5 ounces

Caution Foods	Amount	Caution Foods	Amount
1. oatmeal	½ cup	4. KIND Nut Bar	½ bar
2. plantain chips	½ serving	5. cheddar cheese	1 ounce
3. half-and-half	2 tablespoons	6.	

Sugar-Added Foods	Amount/Calories	Total for Week
N/A	0	200

Recommended Portions

Vegetables: Unlimited low-glycemic options
Proteins: Up to 4 servings per day (4–6 ounces per serving)
Fruits: Limited to 2 servings per day
Dairy: 1–2 servings unsweetened options
Starches: Limited to 2 servings per day
Nuts: ¼ cup per day

Snack Options: 1 serving per day
Added Fats: 2½ tablespoons per day

Download a blank version of this worksheet at EatLiveThriveDiet.com.

Fruits

You should limit your servings of fruit to two per day while you're trying to lose weight or if you are insulin resistant. If you happen to eat more starches than recommended on a given day, reduce your fruit for that day. However, don't make this a regular practice, because the fruit has much more nutrition. Learning to satisfy sweet cravings with your two fruit servings each day is a great strategy.

Proteins

We included four spaces, but you can also add protein to snacks rather than eating another caution food. Including some protein in every meal or snack helps satiate and stabilize blood sugar.

Fats

While we don't ask you to log your fat intake, it does count. We suggest eating approximately two to three tablespoons per day of added healthy fats. For example, this includes butter on bread or veggies, and oils for salad dressings or cooking. We've accounted for nut butters in the nuts category, but no more than one serving per day. Use extra-virgin coconut oil, avocado oil, and ghee for cooking. Use real butter (no margarine) for spreading. We recommend using extra-virgin olive oil for drizzles and salad dressings rather than for cooking because high temperatures may corrupt the nature of the oil, resulting in unhealthy compounds.

Caution Foods

There are six spaces for this category of foods. That does not mean that you should use them all every day. Don't exceed two starches per day. Keep in mind that some of the snack options will count as starch servings. If cravings increase and your energy decreases, that is one sign you are eating too many of these foods. If you gain weight beyond the normal fluctuation of one or two pounds, you are eating either too many high-glycemic carbohydrates and/or too many overall calories. Another possibility is that your body may be expressing a sensitivity to one of these caution foods that you didn't pick up on during your initial testing. We recommended going through the Elimination and Discovery Phases more than once to retest certain foods that could be tripping you up. Keep in mind that this category of caution foods is the most important area to fine-tune. If you are not making progress in your weight loss and maintenance goals, eliminate caution foods as your first defense.

Sugar-Added Foods

If you want the best results for health and weight loss, avoid foods with refined sugar completely. But in a real world, two small servings per week is the absolute maximum you should eat of sugary treats in the portions described below. Sticking with our sweet treats and baked-goods recipes, using small amounts of organic honey or pure maple syrup, is a much better option. And you can eat them daily in moderation as you possibly did during the Elimination Phase. But beware—some of you may respond to any form of sugar in a negative way and may need to avoid it entirely.

Portion Examples
    brownie: 2 x 2-inch square
    chocolate: 1 ½ ounces
    cookie: 2-inch diameter
    ice cream: ½ cup
    pie: ½ slice
    sweetened yogurt: 6 ounces

Approach #2: By the Numbers

This option focuses on monitoring calorie and carbohydrate levels rather than portion control. We'll discuss carbohydrates and calories separately so you can determine the best level of each for you. As with all dietary changes, this is not an exact science, as everyone's body is different. If you are losing weight and feeling great, you are on track. If your energy is low or weight loss has stalled, you will need to adjust accordingly.

How Many Carbohydrates Should You Eat?

To give you a general estimate, most women eat 80 to 120 grams of carbohydrate daily during the Elimination Phase of the diet. As we said earlier, these carbs come from vegetables (unlimited), fruits (limited), and honey or maple syrup (up to one tablespoon). Almost all the women do very well with losing weight and feeling satisfied, so this carbohydrate level can certainly be continued healthily.

If you prefer to notch up your carbohydrate intake a bit, we recommend no more than 120 grams of total carbohydrate per day for weight loss and no more than 200 grams for weight maintenance. Of those, only 40 grams should come from grains or starches, such as potatoes.

Therefore, most of your carbs will come from high-fiber, whole foods, such as veggies. To minimize the possibility of storing excess as fat, do not eat more than 30 grams of *any* form of carbohydrate within a three- to four-hour period. This helps balance your blood sugar and avoid fat storage, which is what happens when excess carbs are consumed.

If you decide to take the "By the Numbers" approach, consider using one of these online resources to count calories and carbohydrates:

- LiveStrong.com
- MyFitnessPal.com
- CalorieKing.com

This is the fastest and most accurate way to determine real values.

There are also many smartphone apps that work well. Find the program that works best for you and use it consistently.

Note that 120 grams of carbohydrate per day is merely an estimate. You will need to adjust the amount based on your own results. Just as you tested each food for sensitivity, test your carbohydrate levels as well.

If cravings increase and your energy decreases, that is one sign you are eating too many. If you gain weight beyond the normal fluctuation of one or two pounds, you are eating either too many high-glycemic carbohydrates and/or too many overall calories.

Weight-Loss Maintenance

Once you've reached your ideal weight, you may be able to slightly increase your carbohydrate intake. Do so very slowly. This is where you risk the insidious creep of carbs and calories, resulting in weight gain that can reverse all your great progress.

Calories Still Count

Adding back many of the eliminated foods—especially starches—will increase not only your carbohydrate levels but your calories as well. If you add 40 grams of carbohydrate per day to your diet, that results in 160 more calories per day. If those carbohydrates are moderate to high glycemic, they are far more likely to be stored as fat and slow down or stall your weight loss.

Calories In Versus Calories Out

Theoretically, if you burn more calories than you eat, your body will tap into stored carbohydrates (in the liver and muscles) and then stored fat to supply the energy deficit. However, the makeup of those calories (protein, carbohydrates, and fat) also influences how well they are utilized. How much and how often you eat also influences calorie-burn efficiency. And as we mentioned, insulin resistance adds an additional layer of complexity to this issue.

The Power of a Reality Check

As complex as this issue may be, awareness of your caloric need is very helpful. Your body is a perfect calorie and carbohydrate calculator. It knows exactly what you've eaten. Conversely, most women are quite inaccurate when they guesstimate their numbers. They often underestimate their intake. So, if you want to be sure of what you are truly eating, counting calories and carbohydrates for a season can be very helpful.

Learn Your Burn

If you're going to take the numbers approach, it is highly beneficial to know how many calories you are burning each day. You can guesstimate this using various online programs. But for a more accurate measurement, we recommend an activity monitor, such as the Fitbit. It will tell you your total number of steps, miles traveled by foot, and total calories burned for most common activities.

How Many Calories Should You Eat to Lose Weight?

Once again, there is no universal answer. It depends on your age, height, weight, sex, and lean body mass. If you've done a lot of low-calorie dieting, your body may not trust you.

It is essential to eat enough calories to support a healthy metabolism. Most experts agree that you need to support your basal metabolic rate (BMR)—the number of calories you need in order to survive—by not eating less than that amount even when dieting. For most women, BMR ranges from 1,200 to 1,600 calories. That sounds high, but it's not.

You can get a fairly accurate guesstimate of your metabolic rate by using the BMR calculator on various websites. Here are two options:

1. www.bmi-calculator.net/bmr-calculator
2. www.caloriecounter.io/calculators/daily-calories-calculator.html

Lose a Half to One Pound of Fat per Week

Slow and steady weight loss is more likely to stay off for two reasons. First, it allows you to make moderate changes that are more sustainable. Second, it supports your metabolism and keeps your body from slowing down in response to reducing calories too much.

By following the recommendations below, you should realize steady weight loss of one half to one pound per week until you reach your goal.

- Eat no less than your basal metabolic rate (BMR).
- Wear an activity monitor and try to walk 8,000 to 10,000 steps per day.
- Eat 250 to 500 calories less than you burn each day.
- Eat no more than 120 grams of total carbohydrates each day.
- Eat no more than 40 grams of starches per day.
- Eat no more than 30 grams of any type of carbs in a three- to four-hour period.

How the Calorie Equation Works

Example #1

    45-year-old woman

    5′ 7″

    160 pounds

    BMR: 1,454 calories

    Steps: 9,000

    Carbs: 120 grams

    Calories burned: 1,975

    Calories eaten: 1,600

    Net calories: +375

This example reflects this woman's *average* daily numbers. Subtract calories eaten from calories burned to reach the daily "net calories" number.

Obviously, the net number should be a positive number to lose weight. A net of +250 to +500 per day is a good benchmark. Because there are 3,500 calories in one pound of fat, this woman is on track to lose one pound of fat about every ten days.

However, if she has a low carbohydrate threshold or is insulin resistant and fails to keep her carbohydrates in check, weight loss may slow or stop.

Example #2

    53-year-old woman

    5′ 4″

    185 pounds

    BMR: 1,511 calories

    Steps: 4,000

    Carbs: 100 grams

    Calories burned: 1,750

    Calories eaten: 1,550

    Net calories: +200

The woman in this example is older but also heavier. That is why her BMR is higher. However, she is also less active than the woman in the first example. She has chosen to eat fewer carbs (100 grams per day) and eat her minimum calories (BMR level).

This gives her a net calorie average of +200 per day. If she stays on track, she should lose close to two pounds of body fat per month.

Keep in mind this varies depending on water weight, bowel regularity, and so on. This woman is ensuring better weight loss by keeping her carbohydrate level closer to what it was during the Elimination Phase.

Other Things to Keep in Mind

As you lose weight, recalculate your BMR with every ten-pound loss. Even though you are supporting your metabolism by eating a minimum of your daily BMR requirement, weight loss means you have less body mass to support. Therefore, your BMR will naturally decrease in proportion to your size.

As you begin testing the "By the Numbers" approach, track your weight, cravings, and energy. If those are changing for the worse, it's time to course correct and lower your calories, carbs, or both. Additionally, increasing activity is often a healthy way to stay on track without reducing your food intake as much.

By the Numbers: Worksheet Directions and Guidelines

This worksheet, as shown in the example on the following page, is designed for you to list the caloric and carbohydrate amounts of the foods and drinks consumed daily. If you like a simpler approach, you can keep a running total of calories and carbohydrates throughout the day, paying special attention to not eat more than 30 grams of carbohydrate within a three- to four-hour period. Quality of nutrition is still important, so here are a few reminders about quality choices.

Vegetables

Vegetables are filling, high-volume foods with tons of nutrients and fiber. Eat them liberally, cooked or raw, and don't be afraid to add some healthy fat such as ghee or extra-virgin olive oil and herbs for flavor.

Fruits

Limit fruits to two servings per day and be aware that some fruits, such as bananas, pineapples, and apples, are about 25 to 30 grams of carbohydrate, which is the most you want to eat at any one time. If you notice your weight creeping up, you may want to eat less fruit.

Proteins

Including some protein in every meal or snack will help you feel satisfied and stabilize blood sugar.

My Weight Today: _166_

Breakfast Foods	Carb Grams	Calories
coffee w/ 2 tablespoons half-and-half	2	40
2 scrambled eggs w/ 1 teaspoon ghee	0	185
1 slice sprouted bread w/ 1 teaspoon raw honey	20	100
1 cup strawberries	11	45

Snack Foods	Carb Grams	Calories
2 tablespoons mixed nuts	3	85
sparkling cranberry drink (recipe)	5	20

Lunch Foods	Carb Grams	Calories
2 cups mixed greens and ½ tomato	14	65
4 ounces grilled chicken	0	135
½ avocado	3	60
2 tablespoons olive oil and balsamic vinegar	5	140

Snack Foods	Carb Grams	Calories
4 cups popcorn	16	130

Dinner Foods	Carb Grams	Calories
6 ounces filet mignon	0	350
2 cups grilled mixed veggies	22	100
½ tablespoon coconut oil for veggies	0	60
1 cup cauliflower mash (recipe)	12	125

Snack Foods	Carb Grams	Calories
herbal tea w/ stevia	0	0

Calories Burned: _1,950_ **Calories Eaten:** _1,640_ **Net Calories:** _+310_

Total Carbs: _113_ **Sugar Calories:** _0_ **No. of Caution Foods:** _3_

Download a blank version of this worksheet at EatLiveThriveDiet.com.

Fats

Don't forget to count your fat calories. Our recommendation is approximately two to three table-spoons per day of healthy added fats. This includes butter or ghee on bread or veggies, and oils for salad dressings or cooking.

Use extra-virgin coconut oil, avocado oil, and ghee for cooking. Use real butter (no margarine) for spreading. Use extra-virgin olive oil for drizzles and salad dressings.

Caution Foods

Even though you are counting carbohydrates and calories, limit starchy foods to no more than two servings per day.

Sugar-Added Foods

It's already been said: less is more! If you want results, 300 to 500 calories per week of sugary treats is the absolute maximum you should eat, ideally in two servings. Watch your portions. These types of treats are highly concentrated.

Some of you will discover that you can't even eat 500 calories of sugar per week without spiraling out of control. This is a strong sign of sugar addiction, and you may want to consider giving up all sugar permanently. It is not as devastating as you may think, and the results will keep you motivated!

Strategies to Promote Lasting Results

Hopefully, you've developed some new (or improved) health habits over the last few weeks. We've listed some of the most important habits and their benefits and hope you consider continuing these as part of your healthy lifestyle. In addition, we've added important discussions on sleep, reality checks, and attitude that we think are essential to your long-term success.

A Lifestyle Reboot

Whenever you find yourself trending toward old habits, do a three- to seven-day Elimination Phase to reboot your body and lifestyle. If you want to test some foods you did not get to yet or retest some foods, we recommend a seven-day Elimination Phase before any new Discovery Phase to ensure accurate results.

This reboot may be all you need to get back in the game and renew your motivation to follow your plan more consistently. As we mentioned earlier, we highly recommend doing the Level 3

Elimination quarterly, ideally at the change of each new season. It's an effective way to stay on top of a few pounds that have crept back and detoxify your body for fat burning and high energy.

ELT Eating Cycle

- Try to stop eating at least three hours before you go to bed.
- Make it a regular practice to fast for twelve hours most days.
- Consider fourteen- to sixteen-hour fasts two to three times per week for the health and weight-loss benefits.

Regular Reality Checks

One of the reasons we gain weight insidiously is because it is easy to be in denial if we don't monitor our body regularly. While we don't want to become obsessed with the number on the scale, that number is helpful in revealing the truth about your fat-burning and fat-storing activities. In addition to weighing yourself, you can also use these alternate strategies:

- Try on a tight pair of pants you've not been able to wear recently and see how they fit.
- Put on your bathing suit and stand in front of a full-length mirror.
- Take your measurements once a month.

Excellent Water Intake

Every cell of the body needs water to function properly. Some of the benefits of good hydration include increased energy, mood enhancement, better digestion, bowel regularity, less appetite, toxin release, and younger-looking skin.

- Shoot for 80 to 96 ounces per day.
- Increase water intake when you drink caffeinated beverages or alcohol.
- Add lemon to your water to help keep you satiated.

ELT Cleansing Drink or Apple Cider Vinegar

Studies have shown that consuming vinegar with a meal reduces the spike in blood sugar, insulin, and triglycerides. It appears to work particularly well in those who are insulin resistant. It also increases the feeling of fullness after a meal.

- Continue to drink the ELT cleansing drink before each meal, or drink two tablespoons of apple cider vinegar in 4 ounces of water before each meal instead.
- Use vinegar as a condiment in salad dressings or other recipes.

Cranberry Drink

- Drink 2 ounces of unsweetened cranberry juice daily to support the body's natural detoxification process and help emulsify stubborn fat deposits.
- Mix with flat or sparkling water and add stevia for a very refreshing drink.

Plan Your Meals and Snacks

Having a plan promotes success. Take the time to review recipes, and make a shopping list at least once a week so you can be sure you'll have what you need. Keep healthy snacks on hand. Consider making several recipes on weekends so it is easy to eat healthily on busier days.

The Journey

We realize that knowing *what* to do is not always enough. Learning *how* to do it consistently is often the bigger challenge. That is why we dedicate ourselves to providing virtual coaching to women who need extra support. We love helping them transform their habits from the inside out.

Weight-loss studies consistently reveal that support and community make a big difference in realizing lasting change. Here are some ideas:

- Invite a friend on this journey with you, and support each other in the process.
- Hire a personal trainer or health coach (in person or virtually).
- Join a community of individuals seeking the same changes you seek.

If interested, you can learn more about our virtual-support membership for women at EatLive ThriveAcademy.com or in the resources section at the back of this book.

A Fresh-Start Mentality

We've said it before, but it bears mentioning again: give yourself grace on this journey toward lasting change. Cut your losses early. Dump your perfectionistic tendencies, and strive for progress.

One of the ways to do this is to adopt a fresh-start mentality. That means that no matter how badly you veer off track, you choose to start fresh every day. In fact, you can practice a fresh start every hour. If you blow it at lunch, start fresh at dinner and choose healthier options for that last meal of the day rather than waiting for tomorrow, next week, or next month. Now is the best time to regroup and reset.

Regular Exercise and Quality Sleep

Both exercise and sleep are essential to your health, weight loss, and longevity. They are so important that we've dedicated a short chapter to each.

Lasting Lifestyle Results Wrap-Up

Now that you've experienced how great you feel when you eat real foods and eliminate those your body cannot handle, keep these benefits in mind as you move forward. Set your mind on your health and weight-loss goals, and teach yourself to love eating healthily. You can change. You can discover a new normal. You can realize your best size, weight, and vitality.

Take time to reflect on all the benefits you've experienced. Whenever you feel tempted to eat foods you know are sabotaging your efforts, tell yourself positive and impactful statements such as these:

- Feeling great and losing weight are more important to me than eating these empty calories that satisfy me for only a few moments.
- I have control over my unhealthy cravings and am learning to crave real and nutritious foods because I love how I look and feel when I do.
- When I veer off track, I make course corrections quickly and cycle back to Phase 1 (Elimination) for three to seven days to regroup quickly and minimize my losses.

Lifestyle Phase
Success Steps at a Glance

- Write down the foods you will permanently eliminate due to sensitivity.
- Write down foods you will limit and consider caution foods.
- Choose your lifestyle eating strategy ("Keep It Simple" or "By the Numbers").
- Drink lots of water.
- Maintain the version of the ELT Eating Cycle that works for you.
- Plan your weekly shopping and menus.
- Have healthy snacks on hand.
- Breathe deeply (see chapter 7).
- Exercise daily (see chapter 12).
- Sleep deep and well (see chapter 13).
- Make frequent reality checks.
- Reset and reboot with a seven-day Elimination Phase as needed.

PART 3

TRUE FOOD

Notched-Up Nutrition 10
Kicking Anti-Nutrients to the Curb

> What you eat (and don't eat) today determines the quality of your health tomorrow. Eat well to live well and thrive in the years ahead.
>
> —DANNA AND ROBYN

In this chapter, we hope to motivate you to take your overall nutrition to a higher level. We'll share the most common anti-nutrients that diminish your health, and we'll tell you about our top ten foods that can help you turn back the clock. Sounds good, doesn't it?

We are bombarded by so many toxins in our environment that it is wise to do what we can to eliminate those we can control, such as in the foods we eat. One of the easiest ways to deal with most of these edible poisons is to avoid processed foods. The less you eat out of bags, boxes, and cans, the better!

Although you can choose to ignore our recommendations and still lose weight through the phases of our diet plan, we strongly believe that long-term ingestion of the items listed in the next section can cause harm.

In fact, if you are over forty-five and have eaten these for years, you probably already experience inflammation and other unhealthy symptoms. Though you may not see or feel the effects of these anti-nutrients yet, your body is quite aware of their negative impact.

Cease-and-Desist Orders

If your body had a voice, she'd issue you a cease-and-desist warning. Because her voice is played out in symptoms and feelings, we're going to step in and advocate for her now!

The following list is by no means complete, but we think it's a great place to start. Consider these as first steps to notch up your way of life and nurture your body.

Keep in mind that when we take efforts to detoxify our bodies, they are much more equipped to metabolize and excrete excess fat. Besides, who doesn't want to look and feel better?

Preservatives and Additives

What you don't taste can hurt you! It is estimated that there are thousands of additives in US foods. Dr. Joseph Mercola lists the following as the seven worst:

1. artificial sweeteners (see page 133)
2. synthetic trans fats
3. artificial flavors
4. monosodium glutamate (MSG)
5. artificial colors
6. high-fructose corn syrup (HFCS)
7. preservatives[1]

It's interesting to note that many additives that are legal in the US are banned in other countries, due to health concerns. We recommend two solutions:

1. Read labels on packaged foods carefully and become familiar with some of the tricky ways food manufacturers hide the truth.
2. Eat less processed food.

Genetically Modified Organisms (GMOs)

Scientists created genetically modified organisms by altering a plant's DNA, making a new species that might contain more nutrients, resist insects or diseases, or require less water so it grows in drought-stricken areas. GMOs were introduced to the marketplace in the mid-1990s. The most common genetically modified foods are corn, canola, soybean, and cotton (which is used to make cottonseed oil).

It is well documented that about 75 percent of processed food sold in American stores contains GMOs.[2] Melis Ann, an environmental scientist, states,

> There is scientific data that shows that GMOs have dangerous side effects in animals. There is evidence, based on animal studies, that eating genetically modified foods causes a wide variety of problems, which makes tracing the source of the problem difficult, especially over time. There is not enough data to show the long-term effects of eating food that has been

Artificial Sweeteners

Danna was a diet-soda junkie from her teens through her thirties. The bubbly, sweet liquid seemed to be the perfect way to get a false sugar fix and fill her tummy without any calories.

Unfortunately, we learned in later years that saccharin, aspartame, and others had many potential side effects. Though manufacturers for products such as NutraSweet and Splenda will boast that their goods are made from natural ingredients, when actually they are concocted in the lab, they produce very unnatural by-products. According to Dr. Mercola,

> Consuming artificial sweeteners like Splenda . . . and products that contain them [such as diet soda] can impair your appetite regulation and cause weight gain. Studies also show that Splenda can reduce the beneficial bacteria population in your gut, increase the pH level in your intestines, and [affect] an important glycoprotein in your body responsible for crucial functions.[3]

A healthy alternative that has been well studied and does not cause this response is stevia. It is derived from a South American herb related to the daisy and ragweed. Studies have shown that this natural, no-calorie sweetener can help control blood-sugar levels.

Other healthier options we like—especially for cooking—include lo han and monk fruit extract. Although neither has been studied as fully as stevia, most experts believe they are good options. Do read your labels, as some monk fruit sweeteners contain other sweeteners, such as dextrose. Depending on how the ingredients are processed, this may make the product less natural.

Some women complain they don't like the taste or aftertaste of some of the healthier sweeteners. Give your taste buds a chance to get used to the new flavor. Patti Milligan has a doctorate in taste-bud physiology and tells us that we sometimes need eight to twelve exposures (or more) to a new taste before we can recognize it as enjoyable. Try the various options, but give them a good chance, as you may discover they grow on you.

genetically altered, but some scientists predict that GMOs are one of the root causes of epidemics that now plague the United States including obesity, diabetes, asthma, fertility problems, food allergies, and even cancer. What about ADHD and autism? There are many conditions that are on the rise which coincide with the introduction of changes in our food system over time.[4]

When in Doubt, Don't

We believe this is a wise position to take when it comes to many of the anti-nutrients we've been discussing in this section, including GMOs. The healthiest solution is to eat fewer packaged foods and choose organic, non-GMO produce.

But let's be real—most of us love the taste and convenience of packaged foods. That's why we need to become excellent label readers.

Read the Labels!

The first thing you need to know is what to believe when it comes to products labeled as non-GMO. Patti Milligan recommends buying only the packaged products that are labeled "100 percent organic" or labeled by the third-party Non-GMO Project. These are the *only* labels that legally guarantee that food is 100 percent non-GMO.

Additionally, to avoid GMOs, buy meats with labels stating that the animals were fed 100 percent organic feed or were grass fed and grass finished (which means they ate grass their whole lives). The same goes for eggs; buy 100 percent organic eggs labeled "From 100 percent organic feed." We believe that some safe grocery-store brands of eggs include Organic Valley, Eggland's Best, and Land O'Lakes Organic.

For dairy products, buy 100 percent organic dairy products (grass fed is even better) or European products from Switzerland, Greece, and France. Some safe brands include Kalona Farms, Organic Valley, Trader Joe's, and Whole Foods' 365 brand.

It's important to note that *most* produce is non-GMO, even conventional varieties, except for corn, radicchio, beets, Hawaiian papaya, zucchini, and yellow summer squash. Most whole grains, legumes, nuts, and seeds are also non-GMO.

Hormones and Antibiotics

Holistic-health and integrative-medicine guru Dr. Andrew Weil states that the US Department of Agriculture (USDA) no longer allows hormones to be used in raising hogs or fowl including chickens and turkeys. However, they are still used as growth promoters in cattle and sheep. Our research reveals that you are much more likely to get hormone-free beef or lamb if you purchase grass-fed products.

Dr. Weil believes that "hormone residues in food may increase the risk of breast cancer and other reproductive system cancers among women, and may promote development of prostate cancer in men." It's estimated that "two-thirds of the cattle raised in the U.S. are given hormones, including growth hormone, testosterone and estrogen, to help boost growth." Producers of beef and lamb may use the term "no hormones administered" on labels after satisfying the USDA that hormones were not used in raising the animals. Dr. Weil recommends that you look for such products if you eat beef or lamb.[5]

Antibiotic resistance is a term that's been thrown around for some time. Bottom line is this: we are exposed to so many antibiotics in our lifetime that the organisms we're trying to kill when we get a bacterial infection are resistant. Sadly, one of our exposures is from the meat and poultry we eat. In an article on Dr. Josh Axe's website, Annie Price writes, "Anything you can personally do to avoid unnecessary antibiotic exposure will go such a long way for your health."[6]

The USDA allows farmers to use antibiotics to prevent or treat diseases in all farm animals, but the drugs must be withheld for a period of time prior to their slaughter so any residue will fall below federal limits. When they satisfy this requirement, they can label their product with the words "no antibiotics added."

Organic Chicken: A Better Choice

To be labeled "USDA Organic," the chickens must be fed a vegetarian diet that does not include any genetically modified ingredients or toxic synthetic pesticides. It also means that antibiotics cannot be used for anything other than medical necessity.

To find lists of farmers known to produce raw dairy products as well as grass-fed beef and other farm-fresh produce (although not all are certified organic), visit EatWild.com. You can also find information about local markets, stores, and restaurants that sell grass-fed products. The Eat Well Guide (EatWellGuide.org) is a free online directory of sustainably raised meat, dairy, and eggs from farms, stores, restaurants, inns, hotels, and online outlets in the US and Canada.

Pork

US conventionally raised pigs are given antibiotics, steroids, and other pharmaceuticals while they are raised for market. In general, pigs are scavengers and will eat their own feces and even carcasses. Other animals do that as well, but pigs' singular stomach diminishes their ability to excrete the toxins effectively, and that makes them more susceptible to viruses and worms. That is why they are given drugs. Pigs also store toxins in their fatty tissue, so when we eat them, we eat those toxins as well. *Oy vey.*

This sounds daunting when all you wanted was that crispy piece of bacon. We personally limit our pork intake and try to choose pasture/free-range pork, which improves the health of the animal and the quality of its meat when we do partake on rare occasions.

Some health professionals believe that pork is a particularly inflammatory food. Studies have shown that marinating pork in vinegar, yogurt, or citrus juices prevents the inflammatory response. Eating bacon or ham cured without nitrates also minimizes the inflammatory response.

Cured and Processed Meats

Salami, pastrami, pepperoni, corned beef, beef jerky, hot dogs, bologna, sausage, and beloved bacon are some of the most popular cured and processed meats. Where do they fit into a healthy diet? They don't. But there are some healthier alternatives that are acceptable in moderation.

Nitrates and nitrites are used in the curing process. These compounds react with gastric acid in the stomach, creating nitrosamines that some experts believe make these foods much more carcinogenic than unprocessed meat. Studies have linked processed meat to colorectal cancer. This includes meat that has been cured, salted, fermented, and smoked.

A study in 2011 found that those who ate the most processed meats had about a 17 percent higher risk of developing colorectal cancer.[7] The World Health Organization (WHO) estimates that a person's risk of colorectal cancer increases by about 18 percent for every 50-gram portion of processed meat eaten each day.[8] Wow. That diminishes your enjoyment of your Sunday-morning bacon and eggs a bit.

There are many products on the market today that are cured with the old-fashioned method of dry salt rub or brine and labeled "uncured" or "nitrate and nitrite free." While this is a better option, we believe that these foods should be enjoyed only on occasion.

What About Shellfish?

In our opinion, shellfish should be eaten in only small amounts. Shellfish are considered bottom-feeders, lacking the digestive system to filter their somewhat toxic diet, which includes some parasites. They are also known to contain contaminants (particularly mercury, one of the most hazardous heavy metals), which can lead to serious health problems.

In addition, most shellfish available in the US are farm raised in Asia in unclean or toxic environments. Some experts consider shellfish unclean and recommend eliminating them completely. This is a personal choice. Be very mindful of how you feel if you eat them.

The Skinny on Fats

Is fat making you fat? Not all fats. It's time to release our fat phobias and identify the good, bad, and ugly fats that are part of our modern-day diet so we can choose wisely. Some fats need to be increased, and others need to be removed completely.

There may be some oils lurking in your cupboards that you thought were healthy but are causing you more harm than good. Those are the omega-6 vegetable oils (such as soybean, corn, and canola), which are known to be highly processed with industrial chemicals. These oils contain high levels of polyunsaturated fatty acids (PUFAs), which are very unstable and easily damaged during processing or high-heat cooking. When these oils degrade in the body, they form free radicals that can cause damage to your cells.

We find the following oils most troublesome:

- canola oil
- corn oil
- cottonseed oil
- hydrogenated or partially hydrogenated fats
- margarine
- safflower oil
- shortening
- soy oil

Got the Munchies?

Some experts also believe that these types of vegetable oils can make you hungry because they contribute to the overproduction of natural fat lipids called endocannabinoids. Notice the similarity to the word *cannabis*? Yep, as in marijuana. Ever hear of the munchies? Excessive omega-6 veggie oils send a signal telling your brain you are hungry.[9] Is it starting to make sense why you can't stop eating that jumbo bag of chips or are hungry quickly after that salad made with a veggie-oil dressing?

Essential Fatty Acids

Both omega 3 and omega 6 are essential fatty acids. This means we cannot make them on our own, so we must get them from our diets because they are essential to our health. These fatty acids play a very important role in heart and brain function, as well as normal growth and development. However, as mentioned, omega-6 fats have been not only corrupted but also overused in processed foods, we no longer need to intentionally add them to our diets in the form of vegetable oils.

According to Dr. Mercola, we would do better to get our omega-6 nutrition from eating seeds and nuts.[10]

On the other hand, omega 3s (such as fish oil and flaxseed oil), which have excellent health benefits, are lacking in most people's diets. Therefore, we need to supplement these because it is difficult to get enough of them in the limited food sources, such as cold-water fish, flaxseeds, and walnuts.

So Less of 6 and More of 3

In earlier times, most humans ate almost equal amounts of omega-3 and omega-6 fats, but we now ingest about twenty times more omega 6 than omega 3. This disparity creates significant inflammation throughout our bodies. If you eat lots of packaged foods such as chips, crackers, breads, frozen meals, and bottled salad dressings, your ratios are out of whack. Ideally, they should be about 2:1 (omega 6 to omega 3).

Improving your ratios can produce benefits such as reducing your cardiovascular risk. Some scientists suggest that your omega-3 blood level is a better predictor of mortality than serum cholesterol.

Add Olive and Coconut Oils

You may wonder where olive oil fits into the mix. It is an omega-9 fat, which is very healthy if properly grown and processed.

Saturated fats such as coconut oil can provide excellent brain nutrition and help you lose weight. You can use these fats liberally in your diet. Coconut oil is linked to improved brain function in many studies and used frequently in natural medicine to improve cognitive function in those suffering with Alzheimer's disease.

Coffee

Coffee has terrific health benefits for some women who use it in moderation and are mindful of its downsides. However, all coffee is not equal. If it is a part of your everyday diet, it makes a big difference what type of coffee you choose.

Conventionally grown coffee beans are among the most heavily sprayed crops on the market. The last thing your body needs is a morning dose of pesticides! Additionally, many pre-ground coffees available at the grocery store are already rancid. Choose organic coffee and look for the "USDA 100% Organic" seal. If you have trouble finding quality organic coffee in your local grocery store, check online, as there are many organic coffees available.

Caution: coffee is a potent substance. When consumed in excess, it can have an adverse effect on your adrenal glands. Listen to your body. Many experts believe that mature women get a greater benefit from coffee when it's taken in the late morning or early afternoon, when cortisol levels are naturally lower. If you need coffee to wake up, you're not getting enough sleep!

Dr. Josh Axe writes,

> It's estimated that 80 percent of people will suffer with some form of adrenal fatigue some-time in their lives. If somebody is struggling with chronic fatigue on a regular basis or has thyroid issues, adrenal issues or hormonal issues, drinking coffee can actually exacerbate the problem. That caffeine is really the main issue with coffee, as it will burn out your adrenal glands because it can be an addictive stimulant.[11]

Listen to Your Body

Robyn is a "fast reactor" and must watch how much caffeine she drinks, but she finds it is a very helpful midafternoon boost that enhances her performance. She opts for a Nespresso espresso.

Danna, although she loves the smell and taste of coffee, recently reduced her total caffeine intake by about 80 percent because her blood work revealed signs of adrenal fatigue. That doesn't stop her from enjoying the taste and smell. She has switched to a quality Nespresso decaf option. She has not noticed any difference in her energy level.

Speaking of Decaf

For obvious reasons, avoid chemically processed options. Instead, look for Swiss Water Process decaf coffees. Or if you're a fan of Nespresso, call the manufacturer, as Danna did, to confirm how the decaf options are processed. (Nespresso is an Italian coffee machine with high-grade coffee that we both love.)

Alcohol

For those of you who enjoy an adult beverage now and then, we hope to give you some information and guidelines that will support your health and weight-loss goals.

We all know of the dangers of alcohol abuse and alcoholism. Some people can handle alcohol physiologically better than others, and certain people groups are known to have more difficulty with alcohol. This is probably due in part to genetics and different body chemistry. Some experts say that genetics accounts for half of the alcoholism equation.

A Personal Decision

We are not condoning or condemning the use of alcohol. This is a personal decision. We also realize that many women of faith have very different positions on this topic. Our goal is to simply give you the facts.

In the spirit of transparency, we'll share our habits so you can see how differently each of us approaches this issue.

Robyn almost never drinks alcohol because wine, beer, and spirits make her feel so poorly. Even one ounce of organic wine leaves her feeling hungover.

On the other hand, Danna and her husband frequently enjoy nice wines with special dinners or an occasional beer with Mexican food. Danna has no adverse physical reaction to modest amounts of alcohol. She almost never drinks spirits.

Neither of us has a religious conviction about alcohol in moderation, but we respect those who do.

Alcohol Is a Toxin

Although there are some nutritional benefits to some forms of alcohol, such as resveratrol in red wine, the toxins in all alcohol do present a challenge to the body. If you enjoy it and it adds value to the quality of your life, finding a healthy balance and choosing wisely is your challenge.

Alcohol is especially toxic to the liver, and in excess, it will cause your liver to prioritize the detoxification of the ethanol over the food you've consumed. If you are trying to lose weight, you need to know that fat metabolism is delayed while the body detoxifies from alcohol consumption. So, for each drink, you are taking a break from fat burning.

Some of the toxins from alcohol are difficult for the body to process, so they are stored in your fat cells for safekeeping. This gives your body one more reason to hang on to the fat despite your efforts. In addition, alcohol causes dehydration and can affect electrolyte balance. Like with sugar, we choose to indulge in alcohol not because of its nutritional benefits but because of the enjoyment it may bring. Therefore, it is important to indulge wisely and in moderation.

Wine

Red wine consumed moderately is often considered to be a healthy alcoholic option by many experts since it is high in antioxidants such as resveratrol, which lowers "bad" cholesterol, helps prevent damage to blood vessels, and prevents blood clots. With white wine, grape skins and tannins are removed, resulting in a lighter color and removing the resveratrol.

Wine goes through fermentation of the sugar and starches found in the grapes, fruits, various plants, and sometimes rice. Ideally, choose from organic options or from local wineries that use fewer preservatives and additives in their wine making.

Dry red and white wines vary in carbohydrates and calories depending on brands. Dry red wines average 3.5 to 4 grams of carbohydrate and 120 to 130 calories for 5 ounces. Dry white wines are similar, with carbs averaging 3 to 3.5 grams for each serving.

Brut champagne wins the health competition with 92 calories but only 2.1 grams of carbohydrate for a 4-ounce serving. In contrast, sweeter wines add up to 2 grams of carbohydrate and 30 to 50 more calories for the same portion.

Beer

Typically, beer is made from wheat, barley, and hops. Most women do much better with little or no wheat, so beer is not a great choice for many of us. Still, there are many gluten-free beers available today. However, though these beers do not contain gluten, even after the fermentation process, they still have some leftover grain-derived sugars and anti-nutrients such as phytic acid. If you enjoy a cold brew now and then, pay special attention to how you feel later or the next day.

Beers have a wide range of calorie and carbohydrate content depending on the type. For the lowest calorie and carbs, choose a quality light beer brewed to decrease both the alcohol and caloric content. These beers can range from 90 to 120 calories per 12-ounce bottle with carbs ranging from 1.9 grams per bottle to 5 grams. In contrast, some stout ales can top out at more than 250 calories and 17 grams of carbohydrate per 12-ounce bottle.

Spirits

Spirits undergo two processes. The first is fermentation of grains, and the second is distillation. Distillation removes the majority of the gluten from most spirits. The process of distillation is responsible for the higher alcohol content.

Many people enjoy spirits with special drinks such as margaritas, daiquiris, and other concoctions that pack in more sugar and make these choices the most dangerous of all. Those trying to save calories and carbs often use diet drink mixes that contain artificial sweeteners and flavors.

If You Choose to Indulge

Sip slowly because these calories and carbs get pushed to the front of the line and are utilized before all the other foods you're eating. If they don't get burned, you know they'll be knocking on a fat cell for entry within a few hours!

It *is* wise to eat while drinking alcohol to send it to the liver rather than the brain and slow its effects. However, alcohol produces a psychological response in the body that lowers inhibitions and therefore makes it easier to justify poor food choices, so make your food decisions before you start imbibing!

Our Favorite Super-Nutrients

There are a few food supplements worth mentioning here that not only notch up your nutrition but also, in our experience, turn back the clock internally and externally. If you're interested in all the supplements we take, pop over to our website designed exclusively for our readers: EatLiveThrive Diet.com.

The Good Oils

Omega-3 Fish Oil

We've already shared many of the health benefits of omega-3 fats, but there are beauty benefits as well. Danna has been taking a double dose of her favorite omega-3 supplement morning and night for more than fifteen years and believes that it is one of the main reasons she has relatively few wrinkles for a woman in her midsixties.

New York City plastic surgeon Dr. Robert Tornambe explains why fish oil is such an effective anti-aging strategy for the skin:

> Omega-3 fatty acids bolster the skin cell membrane of the epidermis. The skin cell membrane is the outer layer of skin cell and it monitors the intake and disposal of nutrients and waste products entering and leaving the skin cell. The skin cell membrane also influences the ability of the cell to hold onto water.... It leads to moister, softer skin, which promotes wrinkle prevention and may eradicate existing mild wrinkles. Omega-3 fatty acids contribute to the upkeep of the skin cell membrane, improving the texture and quality of skin.[12]

In addition to promoting skin health, fish oil is the only thing that completely stopped Danna's hot flashes. This tip has worked for many of our clients as well. And because the brain is about 65 percent fat, omega-3 fatty acids are essential to its health. If we don't feed the brain the fat it needs, it will use what the body has on hand instead. Over time, this can result in decreased mental function.

Coconut Oil and MCT Oil

MCTs are medium-chain triglycerides. Don't let the name or the fact that they are saturated fats scare you. They are worth knowing about.

MCTs are a form of saturated fatty acid that has lots of health benefits that nourish our bodies from head to toe. These fats go directly to the liver and are quickly turned to ketones, which are excellent fuel sources for our bodies and, more importantly, our brains. They are used up quickly and not stored as fat. MCTs also have become accepted in the treatment of Alzheimer's and other brain diseases.

Coconut oil is the most known source of MCTs, as about 65 percent of the fatty acids in coconut oil are MCTs. Coconut oil has become a popular oil to cook with, and we use it in many of our recipes.

Many health experts think it is ideal to get a daily dose of MCT oils and believe the oils can help us

- think more clearly because of the ketones they produce for energy
- maintain a healthy weight
- improve metabolic function and energy
- experience better digestion
- improve mood

Recently, concentrated MCT oil has become popular for getting higher doses of MCT oil into our diets. Robyn has reported feeling much more alert and clearheaded after a dose of MCT oil in her afternoon coffee.

Grass-Fed Collagen and Bone Broth

Collagen is one of the greatest building blocks in the body and is the most abundant type of protein. It helps repair tendons, ligaments, bones, and cartilage and assists in other important bodily functions.

Unfortunately, as we age, our collagen levels decline. Supplementing can support our skin and hair health and promote cartilage and joint health. It also can support the healing of the gut and reduce inflammation. Because of how it supports the lymphatic system, collagen has even been known to reduce the appearance of cellulite, as it helps detoxify the body.

Bone broth contains collagen and all the goodness of glutamine, glycine, and proline to contribute to all the above-mentioned benefits. You can make bone broth at home; it's quite economical. However, use bones from healthy grass-fed beef or organic free-range chicken. You can find our recipe for it on page 223.

Top Five Super-Fruits

These fruits are the best in terms of nutritional value:

- *Avocados* are sometimes thought of as vegetables, but they really are fruit. They are low in carbs and high in oleic acid (a monounsaturated fat), which is known for reducing inflammation. Avocados help lower bad cholesterol and raise the good. They're also abundant in magnesium and potassium.

- *Blueberries* have some of the highest levels of antioxidants. They have nutrients to help support memory and brain function, have anti-inflammatory properties, and have been shown to improve cholesterol and cardiovascular health and reduce the risk of cancer and diabetes.

- *Cranberries* are rich in vitamin C, manganese, vitamin E, vitamin K1, and copper. Of course, they're well known for helping prevent urinary-tract infections. The phenols in cranberries also help lower low-density lipoprotein (LDL) cholesterol levels, aid digestion, and have anti-aging properties.

- *Grapefruit* is known for supporting weight loss and reducing insulin resistance. It also helps prevent heart disease by lowering cholesterol.

- *Pomegranates* also have very high levels of antioxidants. They have been shown to have strong anti-inflammatory benefits.

Top Five Super-Veggies

These veggies are among the most nutrient-dense foods on the planet:

- *Bok choy* is high in folate and vitamin B6. This superfood supports methylation, which helps control healthy gene expression. Out-of-balance methylation is linked to many health problems, such as heart disease, osteoporosis, diabetes, mood disorders, premature aging, and brain dysfunction.

- *Broccoli* is full of antioxidants and vitamin C. It's known for improving immunity and reducing the risk of cancer. It also supports healthy blood pressure and has many anti-aging properties.

- *Cucumbers* contain silica, which helps form collagen and aids in preventing skin wrinkles. They also contain fisetin, which has been shown to support brain health during age-related decline.

- *Parsley* is loaded with vitamins C and K and the mineral iron. It's been shown to decrease inflammation, digestive issues, constipation, skin problems, gas, and bad breath, to name just a few benefits. It also helps boost immunity.

- *Spinach* contains a large amount of beta-carotene, which provides protection from sun damage, as well as lutein, which can promote elasticity in the skin. Low in calories and high in nutrients, spinach also protects the body from free-radical damage, especially in the colon.

You Are What You Eat

Although it may not be realistic to eliminate all anti-nutrient foods 100 percent of the time, you will greatly benefit from being more intentional about removing them from your diet most days. We hope you will find motivation to kick toxic foods to the curb and add in the super-nutrients we discussed. Remember, the body you'll be wearing tomorrow is highly influenced by the foods you eat (and don't eat) today. Just imagine how much better you can look and feel in the months ahead by starting to implement some of these strategies this very week!

One cannot think well, love well, sleep well, if one has not dined well.

—Virginia Woolf

Many of the clients we coach assume that we keep to a perfectly clean diet and never eat anything off the plan. Well, that's not true for either of us! We both enjoy great food and try to stick to our personal lifestyle plans as much as we can. However, there are things we want to enjoy on occasion that neither of us would claim are healthy choices.

For Robyn, that indulgent food is pasta. Danna's guilty pleasure is an occasional (as in twice a year) decadent flaky pastry. Hey, let's be real. Most of us will eat cake on our birthdays and a piece of pumpkin pie (*with* the crust) on Thanksgiving.

To keep ourselves balanced, we try to follow our 90/10—or at least an 80/20—(healthy versus fun food) boundary most of the time. When we occasionally eat something that is not the wisest choice, we pay the price. For Robyn, that is most often in the form of digestive upset. Danna will feel sluggish or see a two-pound increase on the scale. So we cut our losses quickly and jump right back into our personal lifestyle strategies.

Dining Out

Whether you go to a friend's house for dinner or are sitting across the table with special people at a favorite restaurant, eating out is one of life's pleasures. And we feel that you don't need to give that up *even* if you are on Level 3 of the Elimination Phase! After all, there are distinct benefits to not eating at home:

- You don't need to grocery shop for the ingredients.
- You get lots of options to choose from and don't need to make it yourself.
- Your family can eat what they want and you can eat what you want.
- You can ask for special preparation even if it's not specifically on the menu.

Eating out can be a challenge if you're trying to follow a specific plan. We think that by using our tips from this chapter, you'll find it's quite easy to dine out with confidence. When you do, stick to your plan as much as possible, especially during the Elimination and Discovery Phases, so that your testing accuracy is not disrupted.

Become a Picky Eater

Remember the scene from the movie *When Harry Met Sally* when Sally repeatedly customized her order until Harry was wondering, *Who is this person?* She was a person unafraid to ask for what she wanted. So put on your Sally persona and make requests as needed!

Unless you are choosing a restaurant known for its commitment to healthy eating, you will likely encounter foods cooked in inflammatory vegetable oils or laden with hidden sugars and other troublesome ingredients. The simpler the food you order, the less likely you'll encounter unwanted ingredients.

Because eating out is not the primary source of nutrition for *most* women, just do your best and let go of that which you cannot control! We want you to enjoy your life, so make the wisest choices possible and let go of the worry. Bon appétit!

Best Tip Ever

If the restaurant you're selecting has a website, check out the menu in advance so you can arrive with a specific plan of what you'd like to order.

Grains, Grains, Grains

If you are in the Elimination or Discovery Phase, there are creative ways to avoid all grains when dining out. If you're in the Lifestyle Phase and have determined you can tolerate some grains, be aware that it is very easy to eat way too many of these starchy carbohydrates without realizing it. As you recently read in chapter 9, we encourage you to limit your daily grain servings to no more than two per day and be mindful of serving size. This will promote continued health and weight loss or maintenance.

Eating out may be a fun way to include those grain servings, but the quality of wheat and corn products may be less than ideal. If you love bread, don't waste a serving if the bread is not one of your favorites. If you're eating corn products, such as chips or tortillas, ask if they are non-GMO. After your meal, and the following day, look for signs of intolerance. Some women don't have any sensitivity to non-GMO corn but experience all sorts of disruptive symptoms from the genetically modified version.

Favorite Cuisines

We've listed some of our favorite food types with specific recommendations to make it easy for you to stay on your plan. We've also shared a few that can be problematic and therefore should only be enjoyed on rare occasions during the Lifestyle Phase.

American

Salads are always a great option, but watch out for hidden calories and sugar. Many salads today come with dried cranberries or candied nuts with lots of sugar added. Ask for those to be left off the salad.

We encourage you to make some of the dressings in our recipe section (which take as little as two minutes to prepare) and put them in small containers and zippered plastic bags for added purse protection. If that idea doesn't appeal to you, ask for a side of lemon juice or olive oil and vinegar. The next best option is to choose from lighter, vinaigrette-type dressings. Try to avoid those with extra sugar, such as honey mustard or strawberry balsamic.

Sandwiches and burgers can often be ordered in a lettuce wrap instead of a bun. Or just don't eat the bun! You can also ask for salad, sliced tomatoes, or fresh fruit instead of french fries or chips. Broth-based soups are options as well. You can ask your server if any soups contain thickeners such as wheat, cream, and cornstarch.

Or choose from entrées with lots of grilled vegetables and protein such as grilled chicken, broiled salmon, or other fish.

Steak and Seafood

These restaurants usually offer a variety of proteins cooked in a few different ways. You can choose beef, poultry, or fish. Do try to avoid heavy sauces that usually are thickened with wheat or corn-starch. Request extra veggies instead of a potato or rice.

During the Lifestyle Phase, enjoy a half of a potato or a half cup of rice. Pass on the bread (very few restaurants have tasty bread anyway). If you'd like an appetizer, choose a protein or veggie option (perhaps grilled cauliflower) and share it with others. Instead of having dessert, opt for a cappuccino or espresso to finish off your meal. Decaf if it's late!

Italian

Italian food can be a bit tricky depending on the extent of the menu. It's most challenging if the focus is only pizza and pasta. If you don't see many other options, choose a pasta dish that has a substantial protein source, such as chicken. Ask your server to have the cook serve the pasta sauce over steamed zucchini or other veggies rather than noodles.

Many Italian restaurants have fish or lamb options. If they are served with a side of pasta, ask for veggies or a salad instead. Most restaurants are happy to accommodate. Of course, skip the breadsticks and pizza if you're in Phase 1 or 2.

If you're in the Lifestyle Phase and have decided to eat a small amount of wheat products on occasion, ask that the pasta serving be cut to one-half or even one-third the normal serving and don't take home the excess.

Also, if you are in the Lifestyle Phase, remember that one slice of pizza is one serving. Whoa! Most people eat two or three slices. If you opt for pizza, choose one slice and a salad or have a slice and share a protein entrée with someone.

As always, pay attention to how you feel later or the next day. Even if you aren't in the testing phase, many discoveries can be made as you develop your long-term lifestyle eating plan.

Mexican

Mexican is a favorite where we live in Southern California. Being so close to the border, we have some of the most authentic and fresh Mexican food in the US.

One of the biggest challenges Danna faces at these restaurants is that basket of crispy, salty tortilla chips that are served immediately upon her arrival. We think the devil invented those pesky morsels just to torment us. They are so hard to resist! Ask your server for some raw vegetables, such as radishes or carrots, to dip in the salsa or guacamole. No reason you can't still enjoy the condiment and stay on your plan!

While everyone else is munching, you can practice your healthy self-talk by saying something like this: *I can sit here and enjoy the conversation without crunching down on those chips, which are probably stale and full of genetically modified ingredients.* You'll be amazed at how you'll leave the restaurant feeling light and energized, while everyone else is in a starch coma.

Opt for fresh ingredients such as grilled chicken, steak, pork, or fish on top of lettuce or cabbage with fresh salsa, avocado, or guacamole. Choose grilled veggies instead of the rice and beans. Fajitas are always great options, with lots of smoky proteins and veggies. Just skip the tortillas. Eat all the fresh ingredients!

If the menu is limited to things such as tostadas and tacos, eat everything except the tortilla or shell. You may also ask that your burrito or taco be served in a lettuce wrap.

BBQ

During Elimination and Discovery, choose dry-rub seasoned meats rather than wet sauces loaded with sugar. For sides, choose collard greens, coleslaw (this may have a small amount of sugar), or half a baked sweet potato.

Sushi

This option may be a bit more difficult than some of the other choices, but we can make it work. Choose from sashimi, seaweed salad, and salad plates that include fish, cucumbers, carrots, and other veggies. Avoid sauces that contain a lot of sugar, such as teriyaki, and opt for wasabi and tamari (wheat-free soy sauce), hot chili, or, if available, coconut aminos to replace soy sauce.

If you love sushi, you may want to purchase some tamari sauce and carry it in your purse. You can also ask that some of the sushi rolls be made without rice. Remember, there can be hidden sugars in some menu items.

Chinese, Thai, Japanese, and Indian (Lifestyle Phase Only!)

The reason we don't recommend these cuisines for Phases 1 and 2 is that many of the sauces contain wheat, cornstarch, or dairy to add thickness. The sauces also frequently contain sugar or corn syrup as well as MSG (monosodium glutamate), which has been reported to cause headaches and other sensitivities.

It's very hard to know for sure what's added unless the restaurant discloses their ingredients. We want you to get your very best results and test potentially troublesome foods well, so it is best to avoid these options until you are well into the Lifestyle Phase. Then choose these types of food only occasionally.

Real Food, Real Fast

Most fast-food restaurants don't have a lot of options, especially if you are in the Elimination or Discovery Phase. But we've found a few that have better options than most. They are scattered across the US, and we've listed them in the order of how accessible they are to most readers.

Chipotle

This is one of our favorite fast-food Mexican dining options. Not only do they have many non-GMO ingredients, but their burrito bowl can be totally customized to your needs with lots of lettuce, grilled beef or chicken, grilled veggies, salsa fresca, and guacamole.

Panera Bread

Panera uses meat that has been raised without antibiotics. They've taken all trans fats off their menu. However, their ingredients are not necessarily organic or on what we call our "safe list," so use caution when ordering. We like their breakfast sandwich that contains avocado, egg whites, and spinach, and we have it served in a bowl instead of on bread. Most of their salads are good options. Just skip the croutons and chips and bring your own salad dressing.

Rubio's

This popular chain added a healthy component to their menu by including calorie- and carb-conscious items. Order options featuring grilled or seared fish or lobster. Choose a salad with grilled or chopped vegetables, avocado, and chicken, steak, or fish. Instead of having dressing on your salad, choose from their wide variety of delicious fresh salsas. You can also ask for a burrito to be served in a bowl instead of a tortilla.

Elevation Burger

This establishment serves 100 percent organic, grass-fed, free-range beef that is ground at each restaurant location. Their french fries are made with olive oil, and they also offer burgers wrapped in lettuce rather than a bun.

Tender Greens

This farm-to-table fast-and-casual chain has some fantastic options, such as grass-fed beef, sustainably caught seafood, and organic and locally sourced greens. We love the plates that give you an option of fish, beef, or chicken and a side salad. You can ask for grilled or roasted veggies instead of the potato. Skip the bread and you are in great shape with a very delicious plate of food that will fit into any phase of your diet.

LYFE Kitchen

LYFE stands for Love Your Food Everyday. Their beef is only grass fed. They do not serve any white sugar, white flour, high-fructose corn syrup, GMOs, or trans fats. They are a bit pricey at about fifteen dollars per meal, but hey, if you're paying over ten dollars at all the other places and getting lower-quality food, fifteen doesn't seem so high!

Healthy Packaged Foods

Most of us love convenience, especially when it comes to eating. We want to grab something and go. The problem is that most packaged food is full of unhealthy ingredients, such as vegetable oils, additives, and preservatives. It's edible pseudofood that offers nothing more than empty calories.

There are a few options that we eat on occasion. We've reviewed the ingredients and have found them to be as close to real food as if we made it ourselves. Here is a list of some of our favorite packaged foods:

- *Boulder Canyon Potato Chips:* These chips are non-GMO, organic, and cooked with avocado oil or coconut oil and seasoned with only sea salt.
- *KIND Nut Bars:* These tasty nut bars are made with whole food and a small amount of cane sugar. The best option, in our opinion, is the dark chocolate with almonds that totals only 5 grams of sugar, 16 grams of carbohydrate, and 200 calories. Some other options of these nut bars are higher in all three categories, so stick with those that say "5 grams of sugar" on the front of the label.
- *Moon Cheese:* These salty, crunchy cheese bites are made with nothing but cheese! They can be good treats for those who can tolerate dairy.
- *Perfect Bars:* Made in San Diego, these nutrition bars contain organic, non-GMO, gluten-free ingredients. You'll find them in the refrigerated section in a variety of flavors. They average 26 grams of carbohydrate, about 14 grams of protein, and 350 calories. This is one of Danna's favorites. She often eats only half a bar at a time.
- *Popcornopolis Nearly Naked Popcorn:* This is Danna's favorite snack in the whole wide world. The organic, non-GMO corn is popped with coconut oil and seasoned with only sea salt. It can be found in large bags at most Costcos and also ordered online at Popcornopolis.com. (But be careful not to be tempted by all their sugary options!)
- *Sea Tangle Kelp Noodles:* One of Robyn's favorites, these noodle alternatives are made from a sea vegetable. They are gluten free and almost calorie free. You can eat them as crunchy noodles or soak them in hot water, salt, and lemon for softening and serve with a protein and veggie combo of your choice.

A Successful Strategy

Eating out is one of the wonderful pleasures of life. It is much easier than you may think to stay lean and healthy when you have the information you need to make the best choices possible. We've both been on extended vacations to other countries where we've eaten most of our meals at restaurants and not gained any weight—simply by following the tips in this chapter. We also enjoyed many of those areas' special foods but were careful to eat them in moderation.

By choosing the best options on the menu, carrying healthy snacks whether at home or abroad, and simply eating less when the choices are limited, you can embrace the pleasures of eating out without fear of going off the rails!

PART 4

A THRIVING LIFE

What's Exercise Got to Do with It?

Motivation to Get Moving and Tips for Thriving Women

12

If we don't make time to exercise today, we won't have the strength, endurance, and energy to enjoy life tomorrow.

—Danna and Robyn

Do you get winded climbing a single flight of stairs or have difficulty keeping up with your friends on a brisk walk around the block? Have you ever felt as though you're going to collapse from exhaustion after spending the day sightseeing? If your fitness level is so low that you must go into training simply to go power shopping, you need to read this chapter now!

On the other hand, perhaps you've been committed to a regular exercise regime for some time, but your body still isn't changing. You're in the gym three times a week and you know you're healthier because of your commitment, but your body still looks the same. Read on! You may find a few answers to your dilemma.

But if you're a highly active gal who loves to move all day long and you have all the muscle tone and endurance you need to fully embrace your life, then you, girl, get to skip this chapter!

Use It or Lose It

When we participate in regular exercise such as walking and lifting light weights, our bodies are stimulated to build stronger muscles and bones. Why? Because the regular pavement pounding and muscle pulling tell them to get ready for more of the same. They do that by laying down more bone and muscle just where you need them. If you don't use your muscles and bones sufficiently, you'll begin to lose them at an alarming rate, especially if you are postmenopausal.

When we *consistently* live active lifestyles, we're rewarded with many benefits beyond just trimmer and more toned exteriors. Our hearts get stronger, our blood pressure regulates better, our energy improves, and our outlooks often improve as well. Many women report feeling less stress, irritation, depression, and anxiety. There is also an extra benefit of improved self-esteem, mood, and ability to concentrate.

These benefits result in part from endorphins, which are chemicals in the body that give you an "exercise high." The endorphins also help relieve body aches and pains. Danna has realized this personally in dealing with her degenerative back disease.

In contrast, the more sedentary we are, the faster we age and deteriorate inside and out. Lifestyle fitness is about getting in tune with our bodies and making decisions about what we want and need them to do for us.

Our friend Melody began her lifestyle fitness journey to lose weight and get healthier so that she would be around to watch her beautiful little granddaughters grow up and get married someday. This is what she shared with us:

> I'd reached a point in my midfifties where I was feeling decidedly "old." I'd had a hysterectomy, and an old back injury was starting to talk to me a bit more loudly than it used to. I didn't like how old I was feeling, but I tried to convince myself it was normal, even though it didn't feel that way. One day I was playing with my granddaughters and realized that if someone yelled, "Gramma! Go long!" I wouldn't be able to do it. I couldn't even follow them around the zoo for the afternoon any longer.
>
> A year later and thirty-five pounds lighter, I'm a new person. I discovered that it does matter what you eat and how much you exercise. Little things do make a big difference. I began to exercise daily, drink more water, and eat more whole foods. Today I feel ten years younger than the last time we went to the zoo. In fact, my (younger) husband has trouble keeping up with me! I realized that I do have control over things like aging and that can make myself much more productive and energized. It's not about losing weight any longer; it's about maximizing my energy and giving myself endurance and flexibility I haven't had for years. And using my body feels absolutely terrific!

Do You Hate the "E" Word?

Still, women ask us all the time if exercise is essential. That depends. If you hate the "E" word, then your best solution is finding ways to be highly active without engaging in traditional exercise. From heavy gardening and housework to brisk walks, there are many ways to burn calories and work your muscles without breaking a sweat or going to the gym. Whatever you call exercise, being highly active is essential if you want to maximize your health and the quality of your life.

But to take another tack, if leading an active lifestyle is a challenge for you or if *exercise* is a negative word, your self-talk may be sabotaging your success. We encourage you to start changing the messages you're telling yourself. Comments such as "I hate this, but I know it's good for me" and "I can't wait until this workout is over" are *not* going to reinforce new habits.

Write down three reasons you find it difficult to stay active:

1. _____
2. _____
3. _____

Now rewrite those three reasons as positive statements or affirmations. For example, "Exercise bores me" could be rewritten to say, "I enjoy the way exercise makes me feel."

It may seem odd telling yourself a "lie." But it will become real to you when you change your mind by filling it with healthier messages (see chapter 4). And wouldn't it be great to enjoy exercise?

1. _____
2. _____
3. _____

Examples of Self-Talk About Exercise

Here are some healthy self-talk statements that may work for you:

- *I crave activity and find ways to get lots of movement into my life each day.*
- *I enjoy exercise and how it makes my body feel.*
- *I have high enough energy to do all the things I want and need to do.*
- *I engage in aerobic activity four or more times per week.*
- *I park far away from my destination whenever I can and always take the stairs.*
- *Being healthy and fit is important to me.*
- *I work my major muscle groups two to three times each week.*

Being Realistic

There is no doubt that exercise can play a significant role in helping you reach your weight-loss goals, but it's important not to overestimate its contribution. It takes only minutes to consume 500 to 1,000 calories, but it can take hours to burn those same calories off through exercise. If you think getting a good workout means you can eat anything you want in the following hours, think again!

However, if you eat reasonably and increase your caloric expenditure daily by 200 calories per day (a thirty-minute brisk walk for most women), you could theoretically burn off about two pounds of fat each month.

Routines and Resources

Ever since Jane Fonda introduced us to leg warmers and home fitness way back in the 1980s, there has been a multitude of exercise programs available in books and videos. Local gyms and health clubs are easy to find and can fit into most budgets if they're your thing.

> Exercise would be so much more gratifying if calories screamed as they were burned!
>
> —Author Unknown
> (On a plaque in Danna's home gym)

For twenty years, Danna taught aerobics at health clubs and even owned her own fitness studio for a season. After years of working out to music and sweating with other women, she's done with that and finds personal home workouts much more enjoyable.

We encourage you to explore your local resources and find something that meets your personal and financial needs. Our purpose in this chapter is to motivate you to find enjoyable and effective ways to weave intentional activity into your daily life. We'll also share strategies that have worked for us, as well as insights especially relevant to *mature* women.

Exercise Stress: A Gentler Approach

Exercise is a form of stress to the body, and that stress causes it to respond with improved cardio-vascular health, improved muscle tone, enhanced metabolism, and more. However, as we age, we are less resilient and therefore need to be careful not to prompt a cortisol (stress hormone) response by engaging in workouts that are too intense. Doing so can work against us and sabotage our desired results. For example, if cortisol (also a fat-storing hormone) rises, our bodies are stimulated to store belly fat. That is *not* the workout result we want! This is especially true for women who are pre-menopausal and postmenopausal. Frequent, gentle workouts are more effective as women age.

Things some of us did in our twenties and thirties—such as intense aerobic classes, long runs, and high-intensity spin classes—may be too much now, even when we're feeling fit enough to do them. If you love classes with all the energy (and maybe even the competitive spirit), it is important to listen to your body and modify the intensity. Remind yourself that less is more.

These Feet Were Made for Walking

Walking is a safe and excellent way to begin to exercise. It's the most natural activity our bodies were designed to do. It is especially important as we age to wear quality shoes with good arch supports and replace them as they lose their support and shock-absorption capabilities.

Balanced Fitness

If you want your body to sustain you in the decades ahead, it's important to not only live an active lifestyle but also ensure you're addressing all three components of fitness: strength and toning, aerobic endurance, and flexibility. We'll briefly explain their importance and give you some basic tips.

Strength and Toning

Muscles are your body's engine. They are metabolically active, and they burn calories not only during physical activity but also when your body is at rest. Increasing your muscle mass will increase your body's capacity to burn calories. Some studies show it could increase your resting metabolic rate by up to 20 percent. One pound of fat burns only about 3 calories per day. But one pound of muscle burns up to 50 calories! If you gain two pounds of muscle over the next year and nothing else changes, you could lose about ten pounds of body fat.

Muscle tissue without use begins to atrophy within forty-eight to seventy-two hours. As we age, atrophy can occur in as little as twenty-four hours. That is why daily exercise becomes more essential.

You do not have to join a gym. There are many simple exercises you can do in your own home using inexpensive equipment or your own body weight for resistance. We have several of our home weight-routine videos posted on our website LeanHealthyAgeless.com and on our YouTube channel, Lean Healthy Ageless.

Strength training will not necessarily cause you to build large muscles, as women, by nature of their hormones, rarely do this. First, your flabby, untrained muscles will get tighter and take up less space. Then, as body fat decreases, you will notice a nice definition of muscles that appear well toned.

Muscles never turn to fat, and fat cannot turn into muscle, no matter how hard we work out. Fat is fat, and muscle is muscle! If your body still has a fat layer over the muscle, you will not see the benefits of all your work initially. However, beneath the surface, important things are happening. Your increased metabolism and fat-releasing enzymes are increasing the melt rate of fat from your body. You will be seeing some of those toned and fit muscles showing under your skin before you know it.

Aerobic Endurance

Fat burns best during aerobic activity. The word *aerobic* means "using oxygen." The most common aerobic exercises include brisk walking, running, swimming, and biking. Aerobic training causes us to breathe more rapidly and our heart to pump more quickly. With regularity, the body will respond with lower body fat, heart rate, cholesterol level, and blood pressure. Another benefit is increased energy and endurance.

To gain and maintain the most basic cardiovascular fitness, we need to engage in sustained aerobic activity for at least twenty minutes three times a week. This is the bare minimum. Most people need more than that to maintain a lean body.

Aerobic exercise elevates your metabolism while you are exercising and keeps it elevated for some time afterward. The level of afterburn is dependent on the duration and intensity of the exercise. Aerobic exercise also stimulates other systems in your body that burn calories. The result? You become leaner!

Flexibility

Muscular flexibility improves your posture, appearance, and overall performance. By staying flexible, you can decrease the risk of joint injuries and muscle strains. When you have engaged in too much activity, stretching can help reduce muscle soreness. As you get older, your flexibility naturally decreases. However, with a regular stretching program, you can slow down the process and stay quite flexible.

It is important to stretch properly to avoid injury. Ballistic (bouncing) stretching is not recommended; static stretching that holds the muscle in one position is most effective. Your muscles are more pliable when they are warm, so stretching after a few minutes of gentle movement is ideal.

Cross-Training

Cross-training refers to a technique that varies the type and intensity of exercise. There are several advantages to cross-training.

First, the variety allows you to use a wider range of muscle groups, which enhances overall fitness. Second, cross-training helps prevent overuse injuries, which result from doing the same thing over and over. Last, and perhaps most important, cross-training stimulates your metabolism.

Our bodies are incredibly adaptable machines. If we keep doing the exact same thing (such as walking or running each day), over time, our bodies will burn approximately 25 percent fewer calories while doing that activity. So it makes sense to mix up our activities now and then to keep our bodies on their toes!

Dr. Sara Gottfried recommends a little burst training as your fitness increases. She says,

Burst training involves short periods of high intensity exercise with moderate-level exercise as recovery. It is incredibly efficient and comes without the cortisol-raising side effect of a long run. Not only that, but it is extremely effective at raising growth hormone, the growth-and-repair hormone that maintains your lean body mass, a crucial indicator of how your body is biologically aging.[1]

Our Fitness Lifestyles

Consistency and frequency produce the best results. We (Danna and Robyn) have somewhat different approaches that help us stay lean and fit. Here are some of our activities and strategies that have served us well. Perhaps you'll find a few ideas that will work equally well for you.

Danna

- works out in her home gym most days
- doubles her calorie burn by walking at a 12 percent incline on the treadmill
- mixes up aerobic activity occasionally with an elliptical and a stationary bike
- sometimes breaks her routine into two or three ten- to fifteen-minute segments
- does light strength-training exercises five to seven days per week—you can find our arm workout at LeanHealthyAgeless.com or on our YouTube Channel, Lean Healthy Ageless
- practices isometric exercises to develop her core to address her degenerative spine disease
- wears her Fitbit activity monitor most days, with a goal of 10,000 or more steps

Robyn

- puts her workout clothes on first thing in the morning right after getting of bed
- likes to work out first thing in the morning and be done
- loves workout videos such as ChaLEAN Extreme and the Master's Hammer and Chisel—both are from Beachbody and incorporate strength training and light cardio using weights
- does heavier weight workouts three to four times per week
- rides a horse three times a week to improve her core strength
- walks her dogs most days

Tips for Getting Started

- Decide to make exercise a permanent part of your life.
- Set manageable and realistic goals.
- Make an appointment with yourself daily.
- Select activities that you enjoy.
- Incorporate strength, endurance, and flexibility into your routine.
- Try cross-training to maximize benefits and minimize injury.
- Start out slowly and listen to your body.
- Make exercise enjoyable so you will keep doing it day after day.
- Realize that any exercise is better than no exercise at all.

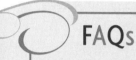

FAQs

Q: What's the best time to exercise?
A: The time that is most convenient for you and when you are most apt to do it consistently.

Q: What's the best type of exercise?
A: While there are many great options, the *very best* one for you is the one you enjoy and will do most often. Walking is always a great option and something we want to be fit enough to do for the rest of our lives.

Q: How often should I exercise?
A: Ideally, daily! As we approach our fifties and sixties, we begin to lose fitness (on a microscopic level) within twenty-four hours of inactivity. If we're not exercising most days, we're moving in the wrong direction. You don't need to work out intensely. In fact, you may not even break a sweat.

Q: What's the best exercise to get fat off around my waist or upper thighs?
A: There is no such thing as spot reducing. When evaluating your body, you are most likely unhappy with the fat that is lying on top of the muscle, and you may feel compelled to do lots of leg exercises or sit-ups. Those exercises are fine for the muscles, but no matter how many times you kick or crunch, the fat is just going for a ride. If you want to see toned muscles, the fat must be burned off. Following Phase 1 of our plan coupled with the Eat, Live, Thrive Eating Cycle is an excellent way to make that happen!

Q: Is it safe for me to continue high-intensity exercise as I age if I'm extremely fit?

A: If you are a woman who engages in long and somewhat intense aerobic or weight workouts on a regular basis, you need to be tuned in to your body for signs of stress or fatigue. You may need a higher carbohydrate intake. This is because your body will deplete your stored carbohydrates (glycogen) during workouts due to high muscle activity. If you feel as if you are losing energy during your workout or feel extra hungry afterward, consider fueling up before your workout with about 20 grams of a high-glycemic snack.

The Irreplaceable Power of Sleep

For Health, Weight Loss, and Longevity

13

Most experts agree that seven to nine hours per night is adequate sleep. Who has time for that? The truth is, we need to make the time. We will sleep well now or we *will* pay later.

—DANNA AND ROBYN

Getting quality sleep is one of the most important components of overall health. There is nothing that can take sleep's place. It is so important that we're dedicating quite a bit of space to this essential health issue.

If you sleep long and well, you are blessed. If you don't, we hope this discussion will provide both motivation and solutions to help you with your sleep issues.

Inadequate sleep decreases the body's immune system and diminishes the brain's capacity for memory and concentration. It also increases blood pressure and overall inflammation and lowers our bodies' pain threshold. The hormones that control our fat cells do not like it when we don't get enough sleep, and our ability to use insulin adequately becomes diminished and creates greater insulin resistance.

Sleep Deprivation

One recent study found that sleep deprivation affects the body's ability to make muscle, as well as causes muscle loss.[1] Because muscles give us the capacity to burn calories, this is the last thing we want. Too little sleep also makes it harder to recover from exercise because it slows down growth-hormone production. Growth hormone contributes to anti-aging and fat burning. We need to do everything to promote that! Also, when you don't get enough sleep, your body produces more cortisol, that pesky old fat-storing hormone.

If all this science doesn't convince you that you need to get enough sleep, maybe this recent study will motivate you. The *American Journal of Epidemiology* published a study that found that women who are sleep deprived are a third more likely to gain thirty-three pounds over the next sixteen years. Getting at least seven hours of sleep each night will help you avoid that outcome.[2]

Snacking and Lack of Sleep

When you give in to that sugary doughnut or gobble up that bag of chips, it's not always about lack of willpower. Lack of sleep affects two important hunger hormones: leptin and ghrelin. When leptin is low, the tummy feels empty. A high level of ghrelin produces hunger and lowers the metabolism, which produces more fat storing.

A recent study found that sleeping fewer than six hours lowers leptin and stimulates ghrelin.[3] Uh-oh. This could be a clue as to why you're giving in to temptation.

So How Much Sleep Is Enough?

How do you know if seven, eight, or nine is your magic number? When you're on vacation or have no time constraints, go to bed and do not set an alarm. Sleep until you naturally wake up and take note of the time. It may take a few days of doing this to realize what your body needs.

If you're not getting enough sleep, chances are you are feeling the effects and may have already tried many remedies. Hopefully, we'll provide one or two new ideas that you've not tried that will offer a lasting solution.

Sleep Disrupters

Not only do we need enough sleep, but we need *quality sleep* as well. Sleep experts say that we go through several sleep cycles each night that include four stages. Each stage seems to have a different job with respect to how our bodies reset, restore, and reenergize. It is recommended that adults get seven to nine hours of quality sleep each night for optimal health.[4]

Sleep challenges can come in two forms: difficulty in getting to sleep, and waking up and having difficulty getting back to sleep. Having both challenges is a nightmare, as some of you know. As we age, we experience new sleep issues and disruptions, especially with the challenges of perimenopause. So let's start with that challenge.

Hormone Imbalance

As women who've had our share of night sweats and early-morning insomnia, we highly recommend that you get your hormones levels checked. An imbalance might be disturbing your sleep patterns. Decide with your health-care practitioner if bioidentical hormone replacement is a good option for you.

Because of extreme hot flashes at night that constantly disrupted her sleep, Danna chose this course for about three years. She felt as though she got her life back. She later weaned herself off hormone replacement and used high doses of omega-3 fish oil to relieve all hot flashes. Fish oil does not work for all women, but it's worth a try.

Caffeine

If you're a coffee drinker, you are probably mindful of what time you think you need to stop drinking caffeine to get to sleep, but you may be wrong. Some people report that caffeine can disrupt their sleep for up to twelve hours.

Alcohol

If you drink wine or other alcoholic beverages at night, it may help you feel relaxed and drowsy initially but could possibly throw off your blood-sugar balance while you sleep and cause you to wake up.

Overstimulation

Our bodies and minds need signals that it is time to start preparing for sleep. When we keep over-stimulating our brains close to bedtime with television, computer work, or even a stimulating novel, we give ourselves mixed messages.

If you struggle to unwind and get to sleep, it is very helpful to create a relaxing and consistent bedtime routine that includes dimming the lights, turning off computers and phones, and engaging in something relaxing such as stretching, deep breathing, and prayer and meditation. Going to bed at the same time most nights is very helpful for long-term sleep habits.

Potty Time

For many, bathroom visits disrupt deep sleep and make it difficult to fall back into slumberland. If this happens often, you may want to consider decreasing your fluids earlier in the evening. If you do this, be careful that you get more than enough fluids earlier in the day.

Sleeping Pills

We realize that some women, out of desperation, resort to pharmaceuticals. If this applies to you, we hope that you will consider them a short-term solution and seek healthier solutions.

Most sleeping pills are categorized as hypnotic medications and can be separated into three types: benzodiazepines, non-benzodiazepines, and barbiturates.

Benzodiazepines—anti-anxiety drugs such as Xanax, Valium, Ativan, and Restoril—help create drowsiness and promote sleep but can also be addictive.

Non-benzodiazepines cause sleep to come on more quickly and allow for longer periods of it. They have less risk of dependency. However, they have carryover effects that can influence your daily activities. Ambien, Sonata, and Lunesta are familiar brands often advertised on television.

Barbiturates are central-nervous-system depressants causing muscle relaxation. They can reduce heart rate, breathing, and blood pressure and therefore have been used to treat headaches, insomnia, and seizures. Amytal, Butisol, and Nembutal are still available in the US, but barbiturates have largely been replaced by benzodiazepines in routine medical practice.

It is interesting to note that healthy people with insomnia often have reduced levels of gamma-aminobutyric acid (GABA). Some sleeping pills work by improving the ability of GABA to bind to receptors in the brain. We prefer the natural approach of using a natural supplement rather than taking a pharmaceutical approach.

Common sleeping-pill side effects include:

- balance problems
- dizziness
- drowsiness during hours when you want—and need to be—awake
- dry mouth
- erratic behavior
- gastrointestinal upset
- headaches
- heartburn
- memory difficulties
- risk of early death
- shakiness
- stomach pain

With these drawbacks, it seems a better plan might be to choose more natural alternatives such as the ones we detail here.

Sleep Enhancers

There is a wide variety of natural supplements that promote relaxation and sleep. You may need to try several of them to discover which ones work well for you.

Magnesium

We both take this supplement almost every night before bed. It helps keep us regular, but there are some other great sleep benefits. In one study, magnesium was found to help reduce cortisol. We don't need a stress hormone keeping us up at night!

By helping quiet your nervous system, magnesium relaxes your muscles and prepares your body for sleep. It also regulates the hormone melatonin, which helps direct your sleep cycle.

Epsom-Salt Baths

Baths are another way to absorb magnesium through the skin. Baths are relaxing and help relieve the stresses of the day, and the salt helps the body release toxins. Fill a tub with warm water, add two cups of Epsom salt, and soak for at least ten minutes.

Melatonin

Melatonin is a hormone produced naturally by the body that helps control your sleep-wake cycles. Your body's internal clock influences how much melatonin the pineal gland makes, and so does the amount of light you're exposed to each day. Melatonin levels start to rise in the mid to late evening, after the sun has set, and stay elevated for most of the night while you're in the dark. They begin to drop in the early morning as the sun rises, causing you to wake up. As we age, our production of melatonin diminishes, so supplementation is very helpful for many. Some experts believe that it also has some anti-aging benefits.

Research has shown that melatonin helps people with insomnia fall asleep faster and improves sleep in perimenopausal and menopausal women. It also creates a calm mood and contributes to increased brain function.

If you have difficulty falling asleep, take melatonin thirty minutes before bedtime. If you are a night owl and want to start getting to bed earlier, take it two hours before your desired bedtime. There are time-release products on the market that are good for those who wake up in the middle of the night and cannot go back to sleep. Caution: melatonin supplements can raise blood-sugar levels as well as increase blood-pressure levels for people who are on medication for hypertension.

CBD (Cannabidiol) Oil

This oil is a compound derived from the cannabis plant. There are two cannabinoids found in cannabis: CBD and THC. THC is the one that delivers the high from using marijuana. CBD does *not* deliver any high at all.

CBD has a calming and anti-anxiety effect that can help those suffering from insomnia mainly because of anxiety. It also has analgesic (pain relief) qualities and has been shown to reduce insomnia in people with chronic pain.

GABA

Gamma-aminobutyric acid (GABA) is a neurotransmitter that can dampen nerve activity. It's thought that maintaining optimal GABA levels may be imperative for restful sleep and avoiding insomnia. Experts recommend taking 500 to 1,000 milligrams before bed for sleeplessness.

Valerian Root

This is a plant with roots that contain many healing properties, including relaxation and sedative effects. It's often found in combination with chamomile in a tea. Valerian root helps increase the amount of GABA in the brain, which helps settle down nerve cells there, resulting in a calming effect.

Teas

There are many herbal teas that have calming properties, such as chamomile, lemon balm, passionflower, and various blends. While these teas may not knock you out like a sleeping pill, adding them to your bedtime routine can be calming and signal to your brain that it is time to unwind and prepare for sleep.

Essential Oils

Many people find various essential oils helpful for relaxation and sleep. The most beneficial include bergamot, lavender, sandalwood, and frankincense. You can rub the oil on your feet or diffuse it and breathe the aroma.

Bedtime Routine

As mentioned earlier, a consistent calming routine and bedtime is important for those who have a hard time getting to sleep. It is also helpful to have your room at a cool temperature. Some women find that a hot bath or shower can induce sleep as their bodies naturally cool afterward.

"Hello Darkness, My Old Friend"

Remember that Simon & Garfunkel song from the late 1960s? Well, darkness *is* a friend when it comes to sleep. The darker the better.

If you don't have the luxury of blackout window coverings, invest in a very comfortable sleep mask. This is especially helpful if you wake in the early-morning hours and want to get back to sleep for your last crucial REM cycle. If you have electronics in your room, power them down. We get enough exposure to electromagnetic frequencies all day long as it is.

Winding Down

One challenge faced by people who have a hard time falling to sleep is the ability to turn off thoughts and stop worrying about the time and about *not* falling asleep. Instead, add a few relaxing practices, such as stretching before sliding into bed. As soon as you hit the pillow is a great time to do box breathing (see page 71) for several minutes. You may want to play some nature sounds or very relaxing music. Shift your thoughts to a time of prayerful meditation or praise. Use a few favorite memory verses that are soothing and repeat them as you intentionally focus on letting every muscle of your body release and relax.

Beauty and the Beast

Body Image and Your Identity

Gray hair is a crown of glory;
it is gained in a righteous life.

—PROVERBS 16:31 (ESV)

Beauty can be both a blessing and a curse. Sometimes the pursuit of it can be like a beast living within us that will not be satisfied when we feel like we don't measure up to "the" standard. Yet who is it that sets our beauty standard? Our culture is obsessed with outward appearance, but who said we had to adopt the same values? Although it is hard to live in a bubble, we would all benefit if we stopped caring so much about how others perceive us.

Think back to your early experiences as a preadolescent, teenager, or young adult. What shaped your thoughts and feelings about your physical body? What messages have you been playing to yourself about your appearance as you age?

> It is liberating to realize that few notice—and even fewer care—that we've gained a few pounds or are having a bad hair day.
>
> —Danna and Robyn

Women in our culture are very aware of the importance placed on outward beauty and are inclined to believe that our value diminishes as we age and our beauty declines. And to make matters worse, many men are more concerned about their wife's or girlfriend's appearance than their own. Sadly, some don't realize that their most innocent comments can be devastating.

I (Danna) had an interesting experience many years ago that illustrates this point perfectly. I had been invited to be a guest on a local television station for a morning health segment. The topic was "How to Conquer Cellulite," and I offered a free pamphlet for anyone who was interested. Over the next few days, hundreds of calls poured in. Later that week, I picked up the phone at my office and began a conversation with a fellow who had seen the segment. The conversation went something like this:

"Hi. I'm calling about that pamphlet you offered on the news earlier this week. I'd like to get one for my girlfriend," he began.

"Okay," I answered. "Did she ask you to get it for her?"

"Well, not exactly. It's just that, well . . . uh . . . I kind of think she could use it."

"Oh, I see," I replied.

"Well, will it work? I mean, do you really have ideas that can help her get rid of her lumpy thighs?" he asked excitedly.

"Sir, there is no magic cure for cellulite. The ideas in the pamphlet can help reduce its appearance if they are implemented consistently. But many women are genetically predisposed to store fat in certain areas. Even some very thin women can still have a fair amount of cellulite on the back of their thighs and buttocks. In general, women were designed to 'jiggle' a little. Is your girlfriend's cellulite bothering her or you?"

"Well, she would sure look better without it!" he answered.

I responded, "May I ask you a question?"

"Sure."

"Is there anything about your physical appearance that bothers you?"

"To tell you the truth, I am going a little bald. That bugs me a little."

"Great!" I replied enthusiastically. "I have the perfect solution!"

"You do?" he asked skeptically.

"Sure! This is what you do. Make a pact with your girlfriend. She'll never look at you from the eyebrows up, and you'll never walk behind her again."

Silence. Not the answer he was looking for.

Beauty and the Bible

As women of faith, we (Danna and Robyn) have struggled with finding a balance. How do we pursue beauty without having it define who we are? We also want to honor God in everything we do. That's why we decided to include this chapter and share our thoughts from a biblical perspective. If you don't share our Christian faith, parts of this chapter may seem foreign to you. Nevertheless, we hope you gain some valuable insights.

There are no messages in the Bible that teach that women must look beautiful or thin to honor

God. However, many references are made to our innermost beings and our hearts. For example, 1 Peter 3:3–4 says,

> Your beauty should not come from outward adornment, such as elaborate hairstyles and the wearing of gold jewelry or fine clothes. Rather, it should be that of your inner self, the unfading beauty of a gentle and quiet spirit, which is of great worth in God's sight.

We see many mentions of beautiful women in the Bible. There's Sarah, Abraham's wife. There's Bathsheba, who caught the eye of King David. There's Rahab the harlot, and Abigail who was praised as both beautiful and intelligent.

It seems that beauty came with its pros and cons. When traveling to a foreign place, Abraham lied about Sarah being his wife because she was beautiful and he feared being harmed because of it. Bathsheba's beauty was a temptation that took David down a destructive path.

There were also times when God used beauty for his own good purposes. For example, Esther, who was called "beautiful of form and face" (Esther 2:7, NASB) was chosen among many attractive young virgins to replace Queen Vashti. By the way, go back and read chapter 2 in the book of Esther and you will find the most extensive beauty regimen of all time. It lasted for a full year and included spices, oils, and cosmetics!

Although Esther's beauty opened doors for her, it was not her greatest strength. Her character and love for her people are most memorable. She was willing to die for others. You may recall reading Esther 4:14 when her uncle Mordecai exclaimed, "Who knows whether you have not attained royalty for such a time as this?" (NASB). And Esther bravely went before the king unannounced, declaring, "If I perish, I perish" (verse 16).

Let's Get Physical—Let's Get Honest

When it really comes down to it, most of us want to be seen as beautiful. As women of faith, we feel conflicted and sometimes wonder if we are too superficial. What better time to delve into our body images than in our mature years, right? It's that time in life when what was once up is now down, what was once in is now out, and what was once smooth is now crinkled. Yet we still care.

If we're blessed to have made it to middle age and beyond, we're living with a painful reality. Our outer selves are wasting away, and we don't like it. We're frustrated and maybe a little angry, because we were created to hate physical aging and death. It was *not* God's original plan. Sin is what contaminated our perfection and caused us to contend with all things imperfect. So in addition to struggling for a lifetime with our beauty issues, we now grapple with the decaying reflection we see in the mirror. What's a girl to do? Run to Scripture, of course!

This is what the apostle Paul writes:

> We do not lose heart. Though outwardly we are wasting away, yet inwardly we are being renewed day by day. For our light and momentary troubles are achieving for us an eternal glory that far outweighs them all. So we fix our eyes not on what is seen, but on what is unseen, since what is seen is temporary, but what is unseen is eternal. (2 Corinthians 4:16–18)

Perhaps the troubles of aging do not seem "light and momentary" to you, but considering eternity, they are. Nevertheless, we must live in these bodies until our final breaths, and how we look and feel will always matter to us. How do we realize a sense of contentment in our physical lives, especially about the things we cannot change?

Paul tells us exactly what to do: "We fix our eyes not on what is seen, but on what is unseen" (verse 18). This doesn't mean we won't care about our bodies or our beauty; it means we will not be obsessed with them. Instead, we will choose to be fixated on Christ and all the many blessings and promises he's given. One of those promises includes a brand-new, shiny, perfect, glorified body like his one day!

> We know that if the earthly tent we live in is destroyed, we have a building from God, an eternal house in heaven, not built by human hands. Meanwhile we groan, longing to be clothed instead with our heavenly dwelling, because when we are clothed, we will not be found naked. (5:1–3)

That is an amazing promise that God makes to his followers. What a blessing to know that no matter how ravaged our bodies become from aging or disease, they will not be our permanent states. One day we will be completely satisfied with our physicality. We will not play the comparison game. We will have no pain. We will experience utter perfection. Nevertheless, today we contend with our discontentment, diseases, and decay.

There is a solution for our temporary discomfort. First, we do our part to take good care of our bodies—our only vehicles for this present life. Second, we renew our minds with truth so that we can find peace and contentment.

Time for an Extreme Makeover

How do you see yourself? Are you discontent with your image in the mirror? Do you compare yourself with other women and find yourself lacking? Do you feel insecure and unattractive and these thoughts disrupt your life? If so, then it's time for an extreme makeover—of your perspective!

You are not alone. At one time or another, most women are discontent with their appearances. They become problems—perhaps even strongholds—when they disrupt their qualities of life. If you think you have good reason to be discontent with your looks, you need to know that many supermodels are the most discontent women on the planet. The more that women rely on their appearances, the more potential they have for experiencing negative body-image issues.

When our self-concepts are warped, it's difficult to let go of what we think we should look like and accept what God designed us to be. This is not to say that it is wrong to desire a leaner or more toned body. It is not wrong to want to be beautiful and even pursue ways to enhance our beauty if we have the means to do so. The key is to put the pursuit of physical improvement in its place and let go of that which we cannot change.

To build a healthy and godly body image, we need healthy and godly perspectives and expectations. We need to see ourselves from God's perspective, not the world's.

Look around you. How many women do you see who look perfect by today's standard? Not many. Just imagine if you didn't pick up one magazine, newspaper, or catalog in the next five years. What if you never watched one minute of television? What would your physical expectations be of yourself? It would be much easier for you to accept and celebrate your body and appearance if you stopped comparing it to an unrealistic standard.

Our lack of contentment comes from deep-seated unhealthy thinking. It takes a lot of negative messages to develop a destructive body image and takes a lot of healthy ones to erase and replace them. If you struggle in this area, give yourself time and grace to change.

As with all areas of life, it is essential to do a reality check before you can move forward. What do you think and, more importantly, believe about yourself? We need to discover the lies before we can replace them with truth.

You will discover some interesting things about yourself from the following questions and exercises that are designed to help you get in touch with your current body image.

- If you could snap your fingers and immediately change one aspect of your physical appearance in any way, what would you change?
- Consider your total physical body in all areas, and list three things you like.
- Was the exercise above difficult to complete? If yes, why?

- Consider all other aspects of yourself, and list three nonphysical things that you like.
- Was the above question difficult to answer? If yes, why?
- Consider your total self, and list three things you do not like about yourself.

Of course, there are no right or wrong answers; you're just doing a reality check on your current self-image. For most of us, the last exercise was the easiest one of all because we're so good at seeing what we perceive as our weaknesses. Although it is not unhealthy to have an objective, critical eye when evaluating ourselves, we need to see our positive attributes as clearly as we see our flaws.

Christ-Confidence

Do you believe that God made you in his image? Rather than desiring self-confidence, we believe God calls us to Christ-confidence, which comes from learning to see ourselves through our Creator's eyes. By taking an inventory of our current attitudes, we can identify our unhealthy thoughts and surrender them to God. We can ask him to help us discard those falsehoods and embrace the truth of who we are in Christ—physically, emotionally, intellectually, and spiritually.

> People look at the outward appearance, but the LORD looks at the heart.
>
> —1 Samuel 16:7

As you review the previous exercises, think about your answers. Do they glorify God? Do they reflect how you *want* to see yourself? Do they reflect how God sees you? If not, change them! Change the negative messages by embracing the truth. Refocus your attention on seeing yourself from God's viewpoint. He sees you as a complete person—body, soul, and spirit. He is most concerned about who you are inside, yet he doesn't want you to disregard your body either. Pray that he will give you an accurate perspective and a grateful spirit.

Try to apply the principles you learned about renewing your mind in chapter 3 to this area of your life as well. Replace the lies you believe with truth. Here are a few examples to get you started:

- *I celebrate who I am and realize I am so much more than just a physical body.*
- *I see myself as a wonderful creation of God.*
- *I choose not to compare myself with other women but instead to celebrate our uniqueness.*
- *I am focusing on my gifts and strengths more than on my perceived flaws.*
- *When I feel insecure or unattractive, I set my mind on Christ and his perfection rather than my perceived flaws.*

It is essential to see ourselves accurately in our completeness as women with both strengths and weaknesses of body, soul, and spirit. There is always room for improvement in every area, but we can choose to focus less on our flaws and more on the fact that we are made in the image of God and that he sees us as beautiful.

Carolyn Mahaney, coauthor of the book *True Beauty,* writes about the beauty struggle:

I can convince myself that I am beautiful for only so long. All it takes is for my scale to register a few extra pounds or to walk past a woman who is younger and prettier than me, and that bubble bursts quickly.

Why doesn't this truth stick? Why doesn't this astounding knowledge—that we are beautiful because we are made in the image of God—eradicate, once and for all, our feelings of inadequacy and self-doubt?

One reason is that we often mistakenly turn this truth about God into clichés about us. When we turn the spotlight away from God and onto ourselves, we twist the truth. So "*God* is beautiful and made us in *his* image" becomes "*You* are beautiful because God created *you.*" Herein lies the flaw in [our well-meaning] advice…: it starts and ends with us.

When we focus on ourselves, we're only compounding the problem. That's because self-focus *is* our problem. Sagging self-confidence is often a preoccupation with *self;* struggles with comparison, measuring up, and fitting in reveal our *self*-absorption.[1]

Carolyn's words are powerful and convicting. If we cut to the core of our insecurities and unhealthy self-image issues, *self* truly is the problem. And the solution is to learn how to shift our focus, not just to better thoughts about our*selves* but oh so much more to the magnificence and perfection of God. That is something worth dwelling on.

Let's decide right here and now to spend more time reflecting God's beauty and letting it shine *through* us than we spend investing in our own reflections in the mirror. The less time in the mirror, the dimmer our image of self becomes and the more beautifully we will reflect him.

PART 5

RECIPES THAT SATISFY

Food is medicine and a healthy diet is a powerful tool for protecting one's health.

—Dr. Josh Axe

These recipes have been designed to ensure that your Eat, Live, Thrive experience is enjoyable. Our participants have told us that these meals, snacks, and sides have made all the difference in helping them stick to their programs. They discovered countless alternative ways to stimulate their taste buds and satisfy their cravings healthily. Their families love the recipes as well.

You'll see that we've noted what Elimination Phase levels (L1, L2, L3) each recipe can be used for. If your level is listed, it is approved for that level. Others will be designated with an *M* to clarify that a modification is needed for that level.

Breakfast and Grain-Free Goodies

Berry Protein Smoothie (L1/L2/L3)

1 cup unsweetened almond or
    coconut milk, from carton
1 tablespoon extra-virgin coconut oil
    or 1 tablespoon MCT oil
½ cup berries
1 scoop high-quality whey protein
½ banana (ideally frozen, very ripe)
2 to 3 ice cubes (optional)

In a blender, place the milk, oil, berries, protein, and banana. Blend until smooth. Add the ice and blend again until smooth.

Tip: Peel ripe bananas and cut them in half. Store them in the freezer in a baggie. Perfect for your smoothies, and no more wasted bananas!

Serves 1. Per serving: approximately 353 calories, 26g carbohydrate, 12g sugar, 21g protein, 20g fat.

Orange Smoothie (L1/L2/L3)

1 cup unsweetened almond or
    coconut milk, from carton
1 tablespoon extra-virgin coconut oil
    or 1 tablespoon MCT oil
½ orange, peeled and seeds removed
1 scoop high-quality whey protein
½ banana (ideally frozen, very ripe)
2 to 3 ice cubes (optional)

In a blender, place the milk, oil, orange, protein, and banana. Blend until smooth. Add the ice and blend again until smooth.

Serves 1. Per serving: approximately 349 calories, 25g carbohydrate, 13g sugar, 21g protein, 20g fat.

Chocolate Banana Smoothie (L1/L2/L3)

1 cup unsweetened almond or
    coconut milk, from carton
1 tablespoon extra-virgin coconut oil
    or 1 tablespoon MCT oil
1 ½ tablespoons cocoa powder
1 scoop high-quality whey protein
½ banana (ideally frozen, very ripe)
2 to 3 ice cubes (optional)

In a blender, place the milk, oil, cocoa powder, protein, and banana. Blend until smooth. Add the ice and blend again until smooth.

Serves 1. Per serving: approximately 348 calories, 22g carbohydrate, 7g sugar, 22g protein, 20g fat.

Tasty Treats for Your Sweet Carb Cravings

The recipes in this section will help satisfy your desire for foods that have a grain-like texture. You'll notice that the sweeter ones allow you to choose either raw honey or pure maple syrup for sweetening. You can bump up the sweetness of any recipe by adding a healthy non-caloric sweetener. One of our favorites is pure monk fruit extract, which is highly concentrated. We recommend 1/8 of a teaspoon for most recipes. If you cannot find it in your local supermarket, we carry it on our web store at LeanHealthyAgeless.com. We also like the packets of granulated stevia and granulated monk fruit organic sweetener, which are great for sprinkling on top of pancakes, muffins, and so on. They are also easy to carry in your purse to sweeten beverages on the go. Another option is liquid lo han drops. Each of these products produces a very sugar-like sweetness with little or no aftertaste. Liquid or powdered stevia is also an option. In most of the recipes, we will give you this instruction: 1/8 teaspoon pure monk fruit extract or sweetener of your preference to taste.

Pumpkin Spice Pancakes (L1/L2/L3)

4 large eggs
1/2 cup canned pumpkin (nothing added)
1 teaspoon pure vanilla extract
1 tablespoon coconut flour
1 teaspoon pumpkin pie spice
1 teaspoon cinnamon
1/4 teaspoon baking soda
1/16 to 1/8 teaspoon pure monk fruit extract or sweetener of your preference to taste
1 teaspoon extra-virgin coconut oil or coconut-oil spray (for pan)

Whisk the eggs with the pumpkin and vanilla. Add the flour, spices, baking soda, and sweetener.

In a nonstick pan over medium heat, melt the coconut oil. Scoop about 1/4 cup of the batter onto the pan to make each pancake. When a bubble or two begin to form or the edges look firm, flip the pancakes and cook on the other side until golden brown.

Serve with Optional Toppings

1 teaspoon organic unsweetened apple butter
1/2 cup fresh berries
1 teaspoon raw honey or pure maple syrup
1/2 banana, sliced

Time-Saving Tip: Make a double batch and refrigerate or freeze for a future meal.

Serves 2. Per serving: approximately 200 calories, 7g carbohydrate, 2g sugar, 13g protein, 13g fat (not including optional toppings).

Grain-Free English Muffins (L1/L2/L3)

⅛ teaspoon baking soda

¼ teaspoon apple cider vinegar

½ tablespoon, plus ½ tablespoon grass-fed butter, ghee, or coconut oil

1 large egg, beaten

1 tablespoon unsweetened coconut or almond milk, from carton

1 tablespoon coconut flour

¼ teaspoon raw honey or pure maple syrup

1 pinch sea salt

In a small cup or bowl, mix the baking soda and apple cider vinegar. (It will get fizzy.) Set aside.

In a 4-inch ramekin (microwave- or oven-safe), melt ½ tablespoon butter, ghee, or oil. Add the egg, milk, flour, and honey or syrup to the melted butter, and whisk with a fork. Add the baking soda mixture. Mix well.

Microwave for 90 seconds or bake at 400°F for 12 to 15 minutes. Allow the muffin to cool to touch, and then loosen the edges with a knife and remove from the ramekin.

Slice the muffin in half and toast in a pan with ½ tablespoon butter until golden brown on each side.

Serves 2. Per serving: approximately 103 calories, 2g carbohydrate, 4g protein, 8g fat (serving size: ½ English muffin).

Apple Pancakes (L1/L2/L3)

3 large eggs

Dash of salt

½ teaspoon pure vanilla extract

1 teaspoon cinnamon

¼ teaspoon baking soda

1/16 teaspoon pure monk fruit extract or sweetener of your preference to taste

1 tablespoon coconut flour

1 cup shredded apple (about 1 ½ apples), patted dry with a paper towel

2 teaspoons extra-virgin coconut oil (for cooking)

In a medium-size mixing bowl, whisk the eggs. Add the salt, vanilla, cinnamon, baking soda, and sweetener, and stir well. Add the coconut flour and stir until smooth. Add the shredded apples and blend until mixed well.

In a skillet or frying pan over medium heat, melt the coconut oil to coat the bottom of the pan. Scoop ¼-cup portions of batter onto the skillet and flatten into a pancake shape. Cook until golden brown, about 60 to 90 seconds. Flip and cook through on the other side.

Serves 2. Per serving: approximately 222 calories, 18.5g carbohydrate, 12g sugar, 10g protein, 12g fat, 9g fiber.

Sweet Potato Skillet Hash and Eggs (L1/L2/L3)

1 tablespoon extra-virgin coconut oil

1 teaspoon ground cumin

1 teaspoon ground coriander

½ teaspoon chili flakes (optional)

2 medium red onions, coarsely chopped

Salt and freshly ground black pepper

3 medium sweet potatoes, scrubbed and cut into 1-inch cubes

½ to ¾ cup bone or vegetable broth or water

4 large eggs

½ cup roughly chopped fresh cilantro

1 ripe avocado, sliced

Heat a large oven-safe skillet, preferably cast-iron, over medium heat. Add the oil and heat until melted. Add the cumin, coriander, and chili flakes. Cook until fragrant, about 1 minute. Stir in the onions and a few pinches of salt and pepper. Reduce the heat to medium-low and cook the onions, stirring occasionally, until they have caramelized. (This can take up to 30 minutes.)

Add the sweet potatoes and mix with the onions and spices. Add the broth or water. Cover the skillet with a lid and let cook undisturbed for 15 to 20 minutes. This will allow the sweet potatoes to steam.

Remove the lid from the skillet. Use a spoon to create 4 "holes" in the hash, and crack 1 egg into each hole. Put the lid back on and allow the eggs to cook for about 3 to 5 minutes to your personal preference. (Alternatively, you can put the whole skillet, uncovered, under the broiler and broil until eggs are cooked to your preference.) Sprinkle with chopped cilantro and serve with sliced avocado.

Time-Saving Tip: Just cook the onions until translucent, about 10 minutes. The flavor is still good, just not quite as intense.

Time-Saving Tip #2: Precook sweet potatoes in the microwave and eliminate the broth or water from the recipe. Reduce cook time to 5 minutes before adding the eggs.

Serves 4. Per serving: approximately 208 calories, 25g carbohydrate, 8g protein, 8.5g fat.

Carrot Apple Pumpkin Muffins (L1/L2/L3)

6 large eggs, beaten

¼ cup canned pumpkin (nothing added)

½ cup extra-virgin coconut oil, melted

1 teaspoon pure vanilla extract

1 banana, mashed

½ cup coconut flour

Dash of sea salt

¼ teaspoon baking soda

⅛ teaspoon pure monk fruit extract or sweetener of your preference to taste

1 tablespoon pumpkin pie spice

2 teaspoons cinnamon

2 cups shredded carrots

1 cup shredded apple (let juices drain in colander before adding to mixture)

Extra-virgin coconut oil for greasing muffin tins

Preheat the oven to 350°F.

In a large mixing bowl, whisk the eggs, pumpkin, oil, vanilla, and banana together. Sift in the flour, sea salt, baking soda, sweetener, pumpkin pie spice, and cinnamon. Mix until well combined. Gently fold in the carrots and apples. Add additional sweetener (if desired) to batter and mix well.

Grease a 12-cup muffin tin with oil, and scoop ¼ cup batter into each muffin cup. Bake for 35 to 40 minutes or until the tops and edges are starting to brown. Refrigerate or freeze extra muffins. These are great for snacks.

Makes 12 muffins. Per muffin: approximately 163 calories, 9g carbohydrate, 4.5g sugar, 4g protein, 12g fat.

Banana Pancakes (Lifestyle Phase Only)

1 small banana, mashed

2 large eggs

½ teaspoon baking powder

½ teaspoon cinnamon (optional)

1 teaspoon extra-virgin coconut oil

½ cup fresh or thawed frozen berries (optional)

1/16 teaspoon pure monk fruit extract or sweetener of your preference to taste (optional)

Whisk the banana, eggs, baking powder, and cinnamon (if desired) together to make a batter.

Heat a skillet or griddle on medium heat. Rub the surface with the oil. Drop the batter onto the skillet and cook the pancake for 2 to 3 minutes, watching for the top to start bubbling. Flip the pancake and cook until golden on each side. Transfer the pancake to a plate. Serve with berries (if desired). Add sweetener of preference if you desire more sweetness.

Serves 1. Per serving: approximately 303 calories, 30g carbohydrate, 17g sugar, 14g protein, 14g fat (with berries).

Berry Goat Cheese Crepes (L1/L2M/L3M)

Crepes
4 large eggs

½ cup unsweetened almond or coconut milk, from carton

1 tablespoon extra-virgin coconut oil, plus 1 to 2 teaspoons additional for griddle

⅛ teaspoon salt

2 tablespoons coconut or almond flour

Filling
6 tablespoons crumbled goat cheese

1 tablespoon raw honey or pure maple syrup

¾ cup fresh berries

Granulated stevia or granulated monk fruit organic sweetener to sprinkle

In a food processor or blender, place eggs, milk, 1 tablespoon coconut oil, salt, and flour. Pulse or blend until well mixed. Heat a griddle or crepe pan to medium-high heat and melt 1 to 2 teaspoons oil to prevent sticking.

For each crepe, pour a third of the mixture onto the pan and move the pan about to let the liquid drain out from the center to create a thinner crepe. Cook until there are bubbles throughout and you can slide a spatula under all areas. Using two spatulas or a crepe turner, flip the crepe to cook the other side.

While the second side is cooking, add about 2 tablespoons goat cheese crumbles on top so the cheese will melt a bit. Drizzle about 1 teaspoon honey or syrup for sweetness. Remove crepe from heat when the bottom is golden brown and slides easily around the pan. Add ¼ cup berries on top, fold over, and slide onto a plate. Sprinkle a small amount of the granulated stevia or monk fruit on top of the crepe (if desired).

Modification: L2/L3—Delete goat cheese.

Makes 3 crepes. Per crepe: approximately 266 calories, 13g carbohydrate, 8g sugar, 11g protein, 19g fat.

Snickerdoodle Muffins (L1/L2/L3)

6 large eggs

¼ cup raw honey or pure maple syrup

½ cup extra-virgin coconut oil, melted

¾ cup unsweetened coconut or almond milk, from carton

1 tablespoon apple cider vinegar

1 teaspoon pure vanilla extract

¾ cup coconut flour

½ teaspoon salt

½ teaspoon baking soda

⅛ teaspoon pure monk fruit extract or sweetener of your preference to taste

1 teaspoon cinnamon, plus additional for sprinkling

Granulated stevia or granulated monk fruit organic sweetener to sprinkle

Preheat the oven to 375°F.

In a medium bowl, mix the eggs with a whisk. Add the honey or syrup, oil, milk, apple cider vinegar, and vanilla. Whisk until combined.

In a large bowl, combine the flour, salt, baking soda, sweetener of preference, and cinnamon. Add the wet ingredients to dry and mix until combined into a batter. The batter will thicken gradually as the liquid ingredients get absorbed.

Spoon half the batter into 12 ungreased muffin cups and fill half full. Sprinkle with cinnamon and non-sugar sweetener, and then top off muffin tins with remaining batter and sprinkle again. Bake for 20 to 22 minutes or until the muffins are cooked through the middle and the edges and tops are starting to turn golden.

Cake Option: Pour batter into an 8 x 8-inch cake pan and cook for 25 to 28 minutes or until the edges and top are starting to turn golden.

Makes 12 muffins. Per muffin: approximately 160 calories, 9g carbohydrate, 4.5g sugar, 3.5g protein, 12g fat (1 muffin counts as 1 teaspoon honey/maple syrup).

Lemon Poppy Seed Muffins (L1/L2/L3)

¼ cup coconut flour, plus 1 tablespoon

¼ teaspoon salt

¼ teaspoon baking soda

⅛ teaspoon pure monk fruit extract or sweetener of your preference to taste

1 ½ teaspoons poppy seeds

¼ cup unsweetened coconut or almond milk, from carton

½ tablespoon apple cider vinegar

3 large eggs, lightly beaten

2 tablespoons lemon juice

2 tablespoons raw honey or pure maple syrup

¼ cup extra-virgin coconut oil, melted

½ teaspoon pure vanilla extract

Zest of 1 lemon

Preheat the oven to 350°F.

In a small bowl, combine the flour, salt, baking soda, sweetener of preference, and poppy seeds. Set aside.

In a larger bowl, mix the milk and vinegar. Add the eggs and mix with a whisk. Add the lemon juice, honey or syrup, oil, vanilla, and lemon zest to the egg mixture and whisk until combined. Add the dry ingredients to the egg mixture and stir until combined into a batter.

Pour the batter into 6 greased muffin cups, filling three-quarters full. Bake for 25 minutes or until they're cooked through the middle and the edges and tops are starting to turn golden. Leave muffins in the cups until they are cool to the touch and then transfer them to a serving plate. Allow leftover muffins to cool completely before storing in the refrigerator or freezer. Great with breakfast or for a snack.

Makes 6 muffins. Per muffin: approximately 160 calories, 9g carbohydrate, 3g sugar, 3.5g protein, 12g fat (1 muffin counts as 1 teaspoon honey/maple syrup).

Spinach Frittata (L1/L2/L3)

½ tablespoon, plus ½ tablespoon
    extra-virgin coconut oil
1 cup chopped spinach
1 cup chopped mushrooms
3 asparagus spears, chopped
¾ cup diced onion
8 large eggs
Salt and freshly ground black pepper

Preheat the oven to 350°F.

In an oven-safe skillet, melt ½ tablespoon oil over medium heat. Sauté the spinach, mushrooms, asparagus, and onion for 3 minutes, until the onion is translucent and the mushrooms have softened. Remove from heat and set aside.

In a medium bowl, whisk the eggs. Add salt and pepper to taste. Stir the vegetables into the eggs. In the oven-safe skillet over medium heat, melt ½ tablespoon oil. Pour the frittata mixture into the skillet and cook without stirring, 2 to 3 minutes until eggs are just beginning to set around the edges.

Transfer the frittata to the oven and bake 12 minutes, or until it achieves a spongy firmness to the touch.

Options: Use vegetables you have on hand, such as chopped zucchini, broccoli, or bell peppers.

Time-Saving Tip: Just scramble the egg mixture until fully cooked and skip the oven baking.

Serves 4. Per serving: approximately 212 calories, 8.5g carbohydrate, 13g protein, 13.5g fat.

Salads, Salad Dressings, and More

Turkey Nori Wraps (L1/L2M/L3M)

Wasabi Cream
1/4 cup sour cream
1/2 teaspoon wasabi paste
1 teaspoon rice vinegar

Wrap
2 nori (seaweed) sheets (large
    lettuce leaves may be used as a
    substitute)
4 slices roasted turkey
1/4 cup shredded cabbage
1/4 cup julienned carrots
1/2 small ripe avocado, sliced

Options: Replace turkey with smoked salmon. If you don't like seaweed, use lettuce leaves for wrap.

In a small bowl or ramekin, mix the sour cream, wasabi paste, and rice vinegar until smooth and there are no chunks of the wasabi paste. Taste it to see if more wasabi or sour cream is needed.

Take a sheet of nori and spread a spoonful of the wasabi cream mixture across a section horizontally. Lay 2 slices of turkey across the nori sheet, and layer with cabbage, carrots, and avocado. Add another smear of wasabi cream over the top of your meat and veggies. Carefully roll up your wrap. Eat it whole, or slice it in half.

Modification: L2/L3—Substitute 2 tablespoons avocado oil mayonnaise and 2 tablespoons coconut milk for sour cream.

Makes 2 wraps. Per wrap: approximately 136 calories, 7g carbohydrate, 14g protein, 6.5g fat.

Coleslaw (L1/L2/L3)

2 (10-ounce) bags of shredded
    coleslaw, undressed

Dressing
1/8 cup raw honey or pure maple syrup
1/2 cup apple cider vinegar
1/4 cup extra-virgin olive oil
1/2 teaspoon salt
1/2 teaspoon dry mustard
1/2 teaspoon celery seed
1/2 teaspoon garlic powder
1/2 teaspoon black pepper
Stevia (optional)

Pour the coleslaw into a large bowl.

Place a small saucepan over medium heat. Add the dressing ingredients. Stir to combine, and bring to a boil. Reduce heat to low and simmer for 3 minutes, stirring occasionally. Cool to the touch. Pour the dressing over the coleslaw. Toss with a serving spoon to coat the coleslaw. Cover the bowl and refrigerate for at least 1 hour or until chilled. Taste, and adjust any seasonings as needed before serving.

Serves 6. Per serving: approximately 162 calories, 14g carbohydrate, 5.5g sugar, 0.5g protein, 11.5g fat.

Carrot and Apple Salad (L1/L2/L3)

1 large carrot, cut into chunks
½ green apple, cored and cut into
    chunks
½ teaspoon finely grated fresh ginger
½ teaspoon cinnamon
Juice from ½ lemon
4 ounces cold cooked chicken breast,
    cubed
Olive oil, for drizzle
Salt

In a food processor, place the carrot and apple chunks, ginger, cinnamon, and lemon juice. Pulse to ¼-inch or ½-inch chunks. Pour into a serving bowl. Add the chicken and mix. Drizzle with extra-virgin olive oil and a dash of salt. Serve immediately.

Serves 1. Per serving: approximately 187 calories, 18g carbohydrate, 10g sugar, 22g protein, 3g fat.

Strawberry Balsamic Chicken Salad (L1/L2M/L3M)

Salad
5 to 6 ounces spinach or other greens
    of your choice
¼ to ½ cup chopped red onion
1 cup sliced organic strawberries
1 cup sliced roasted almonds
¼ cup crumbled feta or goat cheese
2 precooked free-range chicken
    breasts (or 8 to 12 ounces of
    roasted chicken)

Dressing
½ cup extra-virgin olive oil
½ cup balsamic vinegar
1 tablespoon raw honey or pure
    maple syrup
Sea salt and freshly ground black
    pepper
1 tablespoon minced garlic (optional)

Combine the spinach, onion, strawberries, almonds, cheese, and chicken in a salad bowl large enough to toss ingredients.

In a small container with a lid, mix the oil, vinegar, honey or maple syrup, salt, pepper, and garlic (if desired). Cover with a lid and shake well. Toss salad with about 3 tablespoons dressing. Store leftover dressing in a closed container and refrigerate for up to one week.

Modification: L2/L3—Delete cheese and almonds.

Serves 2. Per serving: approximately 536 calories, 11g carbohydrate, 8g sugar, 50g protein, 32g fat.

Rainbow Chopped Salad with Grilled Chicken (L1/L2/L3)

1 small broccoli head, cut into small florets
¼ small red cabbage head, finely diced
1 small red onion, finely diced
1 large carrot, chopped
1 red or orange bell pepper, chopped
1 ripe avocado, cubed
12 ounces cold grilled chicken breast, cubed

In a medium serving bowl, mix all ingredients together. Serve with Easy Homemade House Dressing (page 197), Garlic and Herb Dressing (page 198), or Avocado Dressing (page 198).

Serves 3. Per serving: approximately 243 calories, 13g carbohydrate, 27g protein, 9g fat (without dressing).

Tuna Avocado Boats (L1/L2/L3)

1 (5-ounce) can albacore tuna
1 tablespoon extra-virgin olive oil, plus additional for drizzle
1 to 2 tablespoons lemon juice or 2 drops of lemon essential oil
1 teaspoon Dijon or yellow mustard (optional)
Salt and freshly ground black pepper
Fresh or dried dill or basil
½ ripe avocado
½ cup cherry tomatoes, sliced in half

Mix tuna with olive oil, lemon juice, and mustard (if desired). Add salt, pepper, and dill or basil to taste. Serve on top of half an avocado and surround with tomatoes. Drizzle a bit more olive oil on tomatoes and top with more herbs.

Serves 1. Per serving: approximately 318 calories, 10g carbohydrate, 16g protein, 27g fat.

Easy Homemade House Dressing (L1/L2/L3)

2 tablespoons fresh lemon juice
1 tablespoon apple cider vinegar
1 small clove garlic, minced
¼ cup extra-virgin olive oil
Sea salt and freshly ground black pepper
Dried herbs of your choice (optional)

In a small bowl, whisk all ingredients together until combined, or use a blender or bullet to mix.

Makes 3 servings. Per serving: approximately 120 calories, 14g fat (serving size: 2 tablespoons).

Garlic and Herb Dressing (L1/L2/L3)

2 cloves garlic, minced
2 teaspoons Dijon mustard
¼ teaspoon salt
¼ cup apple cider vinegar
½ cup extra-virgin olive oil
Freshly ground black pepper
    (optional)
Dried or fresh herbs of choice, such
    as herbes de Provence

Place all ingredients in a bowl, and whisk until combined. Add water as needed (up to ¼ cup) to thin.

Makes 8 servings. Per serving: approximately 120 calories, 14g fat (serving size: 2 tablespoons).

Avocado Dressing (L1/L2/L3)

1 ripe avocado
1 small clove garlic, minced
Juice of 1 lemon
2 tablespoons extra-virgin olive oil
Sea salt and freshly ground black
    pepper
1 tablespoon finely chopped fresh dill
    or 1 teaspoon dried dill

Mix all ingredients in a food processor or blender. Add a little water to thin the mixture to a desired consistency. Store in the refrigerator for several days.

Makes 6 servings. Per serving: approximately 81 calories, 2g carbohydrate, 0.5g protein, 8.5g fat (serving size: 2 tablespoons).

Cilantro Fiesta Dressing (L1/L2/L3)

2 garlic cloves, minced
¼ teaspoon salt
1 cup packed fresh cilantro
1 cup packed fresh parsley
¼ cup red wine vinegar
¾ cup extra-virgin olive oil
¼ teaspoon raw honey or pure maple
    syrup
Pinch of red or cayenne pepper, or
    dash of Tabasco sauce

In a blender or food processor, combine garlic and salt and make into a paste. Add cilantro and parsley, and finely mince. Add vinegar, oil, and honey or syrup and blend fully. Add your choice of pepper or Tabasco sauce to taste.

Makes 12 servings. Per serving: approximately 120 calories, 14g fat (serving size: 2 tablespoons).

Caesar Dressing (L1)

1 teaspoon anchovy paste
3 cloves garlic, minced
1 teaspoon freshly ground black
    pepper
1/4 cup lemon juice
2 tablespoons sherry or red wine
    vinegar
1 tablespoon Dijon mustard
1/2 cup extra-virgin olive oil
1/2 cup grated Parmesan cheese
Salt

In a medium-size bowl, mix together the paste, garlic, and pepper. Whisk in the lemon juice, vinegar, and mustard. Slowly whisk in the oil until emulsified. Stir in the cheese. Then put all ingredients in a blender and puree until creamy. Season with salt to taste.

Extra dressing can be refrigerated in a sealed container for up to one week.

Serving Suggestion: Toss liberally with romaine lettuce and additional cheese for an authentic Caesar salad.

Makes 8 servings. Per serving: approximately 73 calories, less than 1g carbohydrate, 1g protein, 7.5g fat (serving size: 2 tablespoons).

Creamy Ranch Dressing (L1/L2/L3)

1/2 cup avocado oil mayonnaise
1/4 cup canned full-fat coconut milk
1 tablespoon finely chopped fresh dill
    or 1 teaspoon dried dill
1/2 teaspoon garlic powder
1/2 teaspoon onion powder
1/4 teaspoon salt
1/4 teaspoon freshly ground black
    pepper
Chopped fresh chives (optional)

Add all ingredients to a jar or container that has a lid. Stir together until blended. Put the lid on the jar and shake to thoroughly combine. Chill for 30 minutes before serving. Store in the refrigerator.

Reducing Tip: Thin out this dressing by adding some unsweetened coconut milk (from a carton, not a can). Not only does it make the dressing go further, but it also reduces your calories per tablespoon.

Makes 6 servings. Per serving: approximately 146 calories, 17g fat (serving size: 2 tablespoons).

Entrées

Roasted Free-Range Chicken (L1/L2/L3)

1 free-range chicken, approximately
    3 to 4 pounds
1 bunch of fresh parsley
1 bunch of fresh rosemary
1 bunch of fresh chives
1 bulb of fresh garlic
¼ cup ghee
Coarse Celtic sea salt
Freshly ground black pepper

Preheat the oven to 300°F.

Chop half of each bunch of fresh herbs finely, discarding the tough stems. Divide the bulb of garlic in half. Peel and slice half of the garlic cloves as thinly as possible. (Reserve other half for stuffing inside the chicken.) In a small bowl, mix the herbs and garlic thoroughly with the ghee.

Loosen the skin of the chicken breast by running a butter knife between the skin and the flesh of the bird. When the skin is sufficiently loose, spread some of the herb mixture between the skin of the breast and its flesh. Take the remaining mixture and spread it on the outside of the skin of the bird. Stuff the remaining garlic inside the cavity of the chicken, and then sprinkle the bird generously with the salt and pepper.

Place the chicken in a covered roasting pan and roast it in the oven for 2 hours. Then raise the temperature to 425°F and continue to roast the chicken for another 20 minutes or until the skin is golden brown. Garnish the chicken with the remaining fresh whole herbs and serve.

Makes approximately 4 servings. Per serving: approximately 190 calories, 28g protein, 7g fat (serving size: 4 ounces without skin).

Using Pre-Minced Garlic
Many of our recipes call for garlic. To save time, you can use pre-minced garlic products found in jars, tubes, or frozen packets. Use the same amount as noted for the fresh garlic. Do be sure to check the ingredients for the pre-minced garlic to make sure they do not include any unhealthy vegetable oils or preservatives.

Chicken Fajitas (L1/L2/L3)

2 tablespoons extra-virgin coconut oil
½ red onion, sliced
2 bell peppers (any color), sliced
1 cup sliced mushrooms (optional)
¼ teaspoon garlic powder
½ teaspoon cumin
2 tablespoons chili powder
Salt
3 tablespoons canned diced green
    chilies
3 tablespoons salsa, plus additional
    for garnish
2 chicken breasts, cooked and sliced
Iceberg or butter lettuce or non-
    GMO corn tortillas
½ cup chopped fresh cilantro
1 medium avocado, chopped
    (optional)

Melt oil in a large skillet or saucepan over medium-high heat. Add onion, peppers, mushrooms (if desired), garlic powder, cumin, chili powder, and salt. Cook until veggies are tender. Reduce heat to medium-low and add diced green chilies, salsa, and chicken. Heat until chicken is warmed through. Serve wrapped in lettuce leaves or tortillas, and garnish with cilantro, more salsa, and avocado (if desired).

Serves 2. Per serving: approximately 305 calories, 13g carbohydrate, 28g protein, 15g fat.

Easy-Baked Salmon over Spinach (L1/L2/L3)

4 (8-ounce) skinless salmon fillets
    (preferably wild)
Salt and freshly ground black pepper
1 tablespoon finely chopped fresh dill
    or thyme
1 tablespoon butter or ghee, melted
1 garlic clove, thinly sliced
½ tablespoon extra-virgin coconut oil
½ tablespoon ghee
9 ounces baby spinach
2 teaspoons fresh lemon juice, or 2
    drops lemon essential oil

Preheat the oven to 400°F.

Place the salmon in an ovenproof baking dish, and season it well with salt and pepper. Mix the dill or thyme with melted butter, and drizzle it on salmon. Bake 10 to 15 minutes.

In a medium skillet over medium heat, sauté the garlic in the oil and ghee for about a minute. Add the spinach to the skillet, and toss and cook it until it is wilted. Stir in the lemon juice. Salt to taste. Serve salmon atop spinach.

Serves 8. Per serving: approximately 263 calories, 7g carbohydrate, 27g protein, 16g fat.

Chicken Sausage Zucca (L1/L2/L3)

2 medium zucchini
2 fully cooked Italian chicken or
    turkey sausages
1 tablespoon extra-virgin coconut oil
1 cup sliced mushrooms (optional)
¼ teaspoon salt
¼ teaspoon granulated garlic
½ teaspoon dried Italian seasoning
1 to 2 tablespoons sliced sun-dried
    tomatoes
2 cubes frozen basil or 2 tablespoons
    chopped fresh basil
¼ cup canned full-fat coconut milk
½ cup spaghetti or tomato sauce
    (optional)

Spiralize the zucchini into long noodle strands, or use a vegetable peeler to make wide noodles. Set them in a colander and sprinkle with salt. Let them drain over paper towels.

Slice sausage into bite-sized pieces.

Melt the oil in a sauté pan, and add sausage, mushrooms (if desired), salt, garlic, and Italian seasoning. Cook until the mushrooms are tender. Add the tomatoes, basil, and milk. Cook until the mixture is heated through.

Add zucchini noodles, and cook for another minute until noodles are warm and al dente. (Be careful not to cook the zucchini very long or it will get soggy and add too much liquid to your dish.) If you want the red sauce option, add the spaghetti or tomato sauce to the pan, then mix and warm through.

Serves 2. Per serving: approximately 300 calories, 16g carbohydrate, 24g protein, 16g fat.

Chicken Stir-Fry (L1/L2/L3)

2 tablespoons extra-virgin coconut oil
1 pound boneless, skinless chicken
    breasts, cut into 1-inch pieces
Salt and freshly ground black pepper
1 red bell pepper, thinly sliced
½ yellow bell pepper, thinly sliced
1 small white onion, thinly sliced
2 small carrots, diced
½ teaspoon grated fresh ginger
½ head of broccoli, cut into florets
3 cloves garlic, minced
1 tablespoon coconut aminos
1 teaspoon sesame oil

In a large skillet, heat the coconut oil on medium-high until it starts to simmer.

Season the chicken with salt and pepper, and add it to the pan. Sauté until the chicken is browned, about 7 to 10 minutes. Stir in the peppers, onion, carrots, and ginger, and sauté for 3 to 5 minutes until the vegetables are the desired tenderness. Add the broccoli and garlic, and cook for an additional 2 to 3 minutes until it reaches the tenderness you desire. Drizzle with coconut aminos and sesame oil and stir. Add salt and pepper to taste. Serve by itself or with Cauliflower Rice (page 218).

Time-Saving Tip: Use prepackaged raw or frozen stir-fry vegetables.

Serves 4. Per serving: approximately 213 calories, 10g carbohydrate, 22g protein, 11g fat.

Lemon Cauliflower Risotto (with Chicken) (L1/L2/L3)

2 tablespoons grass-fed butter or ghee

1 medium shallot, chopped

1 cup sliced mushrooms (optional)

Salt for sprinkling, plus ¼ teaspoon additional

Freshly ground black pepper for sprinkling, plus ¼ teaspoon additional

1 medium cauliflower, riced, or 1 (16-ounce) package frozen riced cauliflower

1 (14-ounce) can full-fat coconut milk

2 tablespoons fresh lemon juice

1 ½ teaspoons, plus ½ to 1 ½ teaspoons lemon zest

¼ teaspoon onion powder

1 ½ cups cooked and chopped chicken breast (optional)

Fresh chopped basil

In a skillet over medium heat, melt 2 tablespoons butter. Add the shallot and sauté until tender. Add the mushrooms (if desired), sprinkle with salt and pepper, and sauté for another 2 minutes. Add the cauliflower, sprinkle with more salt and pepper, and cook until tender, stirring frequently. While cauliflower is cooking, in a medium bowl, mix sauce by combining coconut milk, lemon juice, 1 ½ teaspoons lemon zest, ¼ teaspoon salt, ¼ teaspoon pepper, and onion powder. Stir until all the lumps are gone. Once the cauliflower is tender, pour half the sauce into the skillet, stir, and heat through. Add cooked chicken (if desired).

Garnish with fresh lemon zest and basil and serve.

Save the remaining lemon cream sauce for another batch. This sauce is also used in our Creamy Lemon Chicken with Zoodles recipe (page 206). Sauce can be kept in fridge for 4 to 6 days.

Serves 3. Per serving: approximately 288 calories, 7g carbohydrate, 14g protein, 24g fat (with chicken).

Turkey Taco Lettuce Wraps (L1/L2/L3)

1 tablespoon extra-virgin coconut oil

1 pound ground turkey or chicken

1 teaspoon garlic powder

1 teaspoon cumin

1 teaspoon salt

1 teaspoon chili powder

1 teaspoon paprika

½ teaspoon oregano

½ small onion, minced

2 tablespoons minced bell pepper

¾ cup water

1 (4-ounce) can tomato sauce

8 large iceberg lettuce leaves, washed and dried

1 avocado, cubed

Chopped cilantro or fresh pico de gallo (for garnish)

In a large skillet over medium heat, melt the oil. Add the poultry, and cook it until it's browned, breaking it into smaller pieces as it cooks. When the meat is no longer pink, add the garlic powder, cumin, salt, chili powder, paprika, and oregano. Mix well. Add the onion, bell pepper, water, and tomato sauce. Cover the skillet with a lid, and reduce the heat to low. Simmer for 20 minutes, and then remove from heat.

Divide the meat equally among the 8 lettuce leaves, placing a spoonful of meat in the center of each leaf. Top with avocado and cilantro or pico de gallo. Eat it like it's a taco and enjoy!

Serves 4. Per serving: approximately 231 calories, 5g carbohydrate, 25g protein, 14g fat.

Creamy Lemon Chicken with Zoodles (L1/L2/L3)

2 large zucchini

2 large yellow squash

Sea salt for sprinkling

1 (14-ounce) can full-fat coconut milk

2 tablespoons fresh lemon juice

1 ½ teaspoons, plus ½ to 1 ½ teaspoons lemon zest

¼ teaspoon salt, plus additional for
sprinkling

¼ teaspoon freshly ground black
pepper, plus additional for
sprinkling

¼ teaspoon onion powder

1 tablespoon, plus 1 tablespoon
grass-fed butter or ghee

1 medium shallot, chopped

1 cup sliced mushrooms

1 cup chopped broccoli

1 ½ cups chopped or shredded
cooked chicken breast

Use a spiralizer or vegetable slicer to make your zucchini and yellow squash noodles. Place the noodles in a colander, sprinkle them with sea salt, and let them drain in the sink.

In a medium bowl or large mason jar, combine milk, lemon juice, 1 ½ teaspoons lemon zest, salt, pepper, and powder. Stir until all the lumps are gone. Set aside.

In a large skillet over medium heat, melt 1 table-spoon butter, being careful not to burn it. Add the shallots and sauté until transparent. Add 1 more tablespoon butter, the mushrooms, and the broccoli and cook until tender. Add half of the lemon cream mixture to the skillet, bring the mixture to a slow boil, and then reduce the heat to medium-low. Add the chicken and heat through.

Towel off the squash noodles to remove any excess moisture, and then add them to the skillet. Combine, tossing the noodles into the mixture. Cook another minute, just until noodles are al dente. (Be careful not to cook the zucchini very long or it will get soggy and add too much liquid to your dish.)

Serve topped with sprinkles of lemon zest and salt and pepper to taste.

Save the remaining lemon cream sauce for another batch, or use it in Lemon Cauliflower Risotto (page 204). Sauce can be kept in fridge for 4 to 6 days.

Serves 3. Per serving: approximately 288 calories, 7g carbohydrate, 14g protein, 24g fat.

Salmon or Tuna Patties (L1/L2/L3)

2 (6-ounce) cans of wild salmon or
tuna, drained well
2 large eggs, beaten
1 clove garlic, finely chopped
3 tablespoons finely chopped shallots
2 to 3 scallions, white and green
parts, chopped
½ to 1 tablespoon finely chopped
fresh dill or ½ to 1 teaspoon
dried dill
¼ teaspoon garlic powder (optional)
¼ teaspoon onion powder (optional)
1 teaspoon Dijon or yellow mustard
(optional)
Sea salt and freshly ground black
pepper
1 tablespoon coconut flour (optional)
1 to 2 teaspoons extra-virgin coconut oil

In a medium bowl, mix the following ingredients until combined: salmon or tuna, eggs, garlic, shallots, scallions, dill, powder and mustard (if desired), and salt and pepper to taste. Sprinkle in the flour and mix well. If there's still a lot of liquid, add a little more flour, one teaspoon at a time.

In a medium frying pan over medium heat, melt the oil.

Scoop the fish mixture into your hand and form it into a patty. (It should yield 7 to 9 patties.) Place 3 to 4 patties in the pan, depending on the size of your pan. Cook them until they are golden brown on one side, approximately 2 to 3 minutes. Flip patties and cook on the other side until they're golden brown. Place patties on a serving plate and cover until all patties are cooked and ready to serve.

Serving Suggestion: These are great served with Avocado Dressing (page 198).

Serves 3. Per serving: approximately 198 calories, 1g carbohydrate, 30g protein, 11g fat.

South of the Border Stuffed Peppers (L1/L2M/L3M)

2 large bell peppers (any color), halved with seeds and core removed

½ pound cooked or roasted chicken

½ small onion, chopped

1 clove garlic, minced

½ teaspoon cumin

½ teaspoon chili powder

¼ teaspoon salt

¼ teaspoon freshly ground black pepper

2 tablespoons tomato paste

6 tablespoons water

1 (4-ounce) can diced green chilies

½ cup canned black beans, drained and rinsed

1 cup fresh or frozen corn

Mexican-style hot sauce (Cholula, Tapatío)

1 cup riced cauliflower

(Lifestyle Phase Option: 1 cup cooked rice instead of the riced cauliflower—will increase calories by 60 and carbohydrate grams by 13)

¼ cup salsa verde

½ cup shredded cheddar cheese

Preheat the oven to 400°F.

Fill a medium pot with water, and bring it to a boil. Add the pepper halves and continue to boil for 5 minutes. Drain and place the peppers cut-side down on a paper towel.

In a medium bowl, mix together the chicken, onion, garlic, cumin, chili powder, salt, pepper, tomato paste, water, chilies, beans, corn, hot sauce to taste, and riced cauliflower or cooked rice.

Spoon stuffing mixture into each drained pepper half. Place peppers in an 8 x 8-inch baking dish. Top them with salsa. Cover the baking dish with aluminum foil, and bake for 30 minutes. Remove the foil, and top the peppers with the cheese. Return the uncovered baking dish to the oven for an additional 7 to 10 minutes, or until the cheese is bubbling and just starting to turn golden in spots.

Time-Saving Tip: Coarsely chop peppers. In a large skillet, melt 1 tablespoon coconut oil over medium heat. Sauté the peppers with onion, garlic, riced cauliflower, and corn until soft. Add the remaining spices, beans, cooked chicken, salsa, tomato paste, and water. Combine well. Reduce heat to low and simmer until warmed through. Add hot sauce to taste, and top with shredded cheese.

Modification: L2/L3—Delete corn, beans, and cheese, substituting with 1 ½ cups diced carrots and/or zucchini.

Makes 4 peppers. Per pepper: approximately 296 calories, 22g carbohydrate, 21g protein, 14g fat.

Roasted Italian Stuffed Peppers (L1/L2/L3)

2 bell peppers (any color), halved
    with seeds and core removed
1 tablespoon extra-virgin coconut oil
½ large onion, diced
Sea salt and freshly ground black
    pepper
4 cloves garlic, minced
1 carrot, shredded or diced
1 pound ground turkey or chicken
2 to 3 tablespoons tomato paste
6 fresh basil leaves, finely chopped,
    plus extra for garnish
1 cup fresh or frozen chopped spinach

Preheat the oven to 400°F.

Fill a medium pot with water, and bring it to a boil. Add the pepper halves and continue to boil for 5 minutes. Drain and place the peppers cut-side down on a paper towel.

In a large sauté pan over medium-high heat, melt the oil. Add the onion, and cook it until it is translucent. Season with salt and pepper. Add the garlic and carrot, reduce the heat to low, and let simmer for a few minutes.

Increase the heat to medium-high, add the poultry, and cook through completely. Add the tomato paste and stir through. (You may need to add 2 to 4 tablespoons water if the mixture is too thick.) Add additional salt and pepper to taste. Add the basil and spinach, and allow them to wilt. Combine evenly.

Spoon stuffing mixture into each drained pepper half. Place in an 8 x 8-inch baking dish and bake in the oven for 15 to 20 minutes. Garnish with fresh basil.

These go well with Cauliflower Mash as a side (page 219). Stuffed Peppers refrigerate and freeze well and are great for lunch too!

Makes 4 peppers. Per pepper: approximately 242 calories, 6.5g carbohydrate, 23g protein, 9.5g fat.

Busy-Woman Greek Chicken (L1/L2/L3)

1 whole pre-roasted chicken
½ cup extra-virgin olive oil
½ cup fresh lemon juice
4 teaspoons chopped fresh garlic
2 tablespoons apple cider vinegar
Zest of 1 lemon
½ teaspoon salt
Dash of freshly ground black pepper
2 teaspoons herbes de Provence,
    Italian seasoning, or other green-
    herb seasoning, plus additional for
    sprinkling

Preheat the oven to 350°F.

Carve the chicken breast and thigh in thick slices, and place them in an 8 x 13-inch baking dish. Add the wings and legs to the baking dish alongside the other chicken pieces.

In a bowl or jar that has a lid, place oil, lemon juice, garlic, vinegar, zest, salt, pepper, and herbs. Mix well.

Sprinkle some additional dried herbs over the top of the chicken, and then pour the marinade over the top to cover the chicken. Cover the baking dish with foil. Bake it in the oven for 15 to 20 minutes, until chicken is heated through and sauce is bubbling.

Serve with a salad and/or roasted veggies and maybe a few roasted potatoes. *Opa!*

Serves 5. Per serving: approximately 350 calories, 23g protein, 28.5g fat.

Creamy Chicken Spaghetti Squash (L1/L2/L3)

1 large spaghetti squash

2 tablespoons ghee or extra-virgin coconut oil

1 to 2 teaspoons fresh minced garlic

2 large shallots, thinly sliced

4 tablespoons julienned sun-dried tomatoes packed in olive oil

½ cup chopped mushrooms (optional)

1 pound chicken breast (boneless, skinless), diced small

½ teaspoon salt, plus additional

½ teaspoon red pepper flakes (optional)

1 teaspoon dried basil

½ cup canned full-fat coconut milk

½ to 1 cup chicken-bone broth or veggie broth

1 teaspoon sea salt

Freshly ground black pepper

Preheat the oven to 400°F.

Cut spaghetti squash in half lengthwise, discard seeds, and place facedown on a baking sheet. Bake for 45 to 55 minutes, until threads are easily removed from the squash. (Or, in a microwave-safe dish, place the squash facedown and cook for 12 minutes.)

Place a large sauté pan over medium-low heat. Add the ghee or oil (or a combination of the two) to the pan. Once the oil is warm, add the garlic and shallots. Cook until the garlic becomes fragrant. Add the tomatoes and mushrooms (if desired), and cook for 5 minutes. Remove mixture and set it aside on a plate.

Return the skillet to the stove top, add the chicken, sprinkle with the salt, red pepper flakes (if desired), and basil. Brown the chicken on all sides, and add the tomato mixture back into the pan with the chicken. Pour in the milk, ½ cup broth, and sea salt. Mix well. Add in the spaghetti squash threads, and mix until well combined. Turn the heat to low, and let the mixture simmer for about 8 to 10 minutes, or until it reduces and thickens. If it is too thick, add more broth to thin. Add salt and pepper to taste.

Time-Saving Tip: Use pulled chicken from a roast chicken that you purchased precooked or made earlier in the week. Warm chicken through instead of browning on all sides.

Serves 4. Per serving: approximately 334 calories, 19g carbohydrate, 27g protein, 17g fat.

Chicken Marsala (L1)

1 medium white or yellow onion,
    sliced
1 to 2 teaspoons minced fresh garlic
1 cup sliced mushrooms
2 to 3 tablespoons, plus 2 to 3
    tablespoons extra-virgin coconut
    or avocado oil
Sea salt and freshly ground black
    pepper
4 chicken breast cutlets (or 1 pound
    full boneless chicken breasts
    pounded to 1/4 inch thickness)
1/2 cup arrowroot (you won't use all of
    this, but you need enough for
    shaking in a bag)
1/2 cup tapioca flour (you won't use all
    of this, but you need enough for
    shaking in a bag)
Herbes de Provence
1 cup marsala wine
Garlic powder

In a large skillet over medium-high heat, sauté the onion, garlic, and mushrooms in 2 to 3 tablespoons oil. Cook until the onion is caramelized. Remove from heat, and place the mixture in a small bowl.

Lightly shake salt and pepper (to taste) directly onto chicken breast. In a large ziplock baggie, mix arrowroot, flour, more salt and pepper, and herbes de Provence. Toss chicken into baggie, close, and shake well.

In the same skillet over medium heat, sauté the floured chicken in 2 to 3 tablespoons oil until it is golden brown on both sides, about 15 minutes total. Slowly pour in about half of the wine, and turn the heat down to a simmer for about 5 minutes. Note that the alcohol will burn off.

Add the onion and mushrooms to the chicken. Pour the remaining wine over all the ingredients. Cover with a lid and simmer for 10 minutes. Add garlic powder and more salt to taste as the sauce thickens slightly while simmering.

Serve beside or over your choice of veggies, such as zucchini or Cauliflower Mash (recipe on page 219). Mashed sweet potatoes are also nice if you want a few more carbohydrates with the meal.

Serves 4. Per serving: approximately 368 calories, 18g carbohydrate, 22g protein, 18g fat.

Mediterranean Tuna (L1M/L2M/L3M)

1 medium yellow onion, diced

2 to 3 tablespoons avocado oil or extra-virgin coconut oil

1 to 2 teaspoons minced garlic

1 (12-ounce) can albacore tuna packed in water

1 (32-ounce) can stewed tomatoes, well chopped and with liquid

2 to 3 tablespoons capers (from jar)

½ cup diced black or kalamata olives

½ cup chopped sun-dried tomatoes (optional)

In a medium pan over medium heat, sauté onion in 2 to 3 tablespoons oil until it turns golden brown and then stir in the garlic. Flake the tuna into small pieces with a knife or fork, and add it to the sauté pan. Add the stewed tomatoes, capers, and olives. Add sun-dried tomatoes (if desired). Simmer for 5 minutes. You can stir rice, penne, kelp noodles, or spaghetti squash into this tuna mixture for a complete meal.

Serves 8. Penne Option per serving: approximately 221 calories, 27g carbohydrate, 13g protein, 7g fat. Kelp Noodle Option per serving: approximately 124 calories, 5g carbohydrate, 11g protein, 6g fat. Spaghetti Squash Option per serving: approximately 143 calories, 9g carbohydrate, 11.5g protein, 6.5g fat.

Serving Options for the Mediterranean Tuna

Brown Rice or Penne (LS): Use 8 ounces cooked brown rice or cook 6 ounces gluten-free penne pasta according to the package directions. Stir the rice or drained pasta into the tuna mixture and simmer for one additional minute.

Kelp Noodles (L1/L2/L3 and LS): Use 1 (12-ounce) package kelp noodles for a grain-free option. To soften noodles, place them in a colander and rinse them with water. Transfer the noodles to a large bowl, and cover them with very hot water. Add ½ tablespoon salt and the juice of a whole medium-size lemon. Stir for about 10 seconds, until the salt dissolves. Let them sit for 30 minutes to soften. Drain the noodles, and stir them into the tuna mixture.

Spaghetti Squash (L1/L2/L3 and LS): Preheat the oven to 400°F. Cut 1 large spaghetti squash in half lengthwise, discard seeds, and place cut-side down on a baking sheet. Bake for 45 to 55 minutes, until threads are easily removed from the squash. (Optional microwave cooking option: In a microwave-safe dish, place squash cut-side down and cook in microwave for 12 minutes.) Remove squash threads from skin with a fork, stir them into the tuna mixture, and simmer for 1 additional minute.

Ceviche (L1/L2/L3)

Be prepared for this recipe to take at least 30 minutes of preparation time. Prep can be done one day ahead. (The ceviche will stay good 2 days in the refrigerator.) Read through all the instructions before you begin.

1¼ pounds raw white fish (cod, grouper, sea bass, sole, snapper, tilapia), chopped into ½-inch squares
5 medium limes, cut in half
10 medium lemons, cut in half
2 to 3 garlic cloves, roughly chopped
2 jalapeños, seeds removed, roughly chopped (wear rubber gloves when handling)
1 tablespoon extra-virgin olive oil
3 cucumbers, diced
6 firm vine-ripened tomatoes, diced
1 large red onion, diced
2 teaspoons salt, plus additional
1 bunch of cilantro, finely chopped
2 avocados, diced (optional)
Tamari (optional)
Coconut aminos (optional)

Place the fish in a deep bowl. Using a hand citrus press, squeeze 4 of the limes and 9 lemons over the fish. Make sure the fish is fully covered in juice. Cover the bowl and place it in the refrigerator for 45 to 60 minutes. Various fish types cure at different rates, so leave it soaking longer if needed. Fish that appears fully white and pulls apart easily is ready to eat.

In a food processor, gently pulse the garlic, jalapeños, and oil until well combined. Set it aside to add to the final mixture.

Remove the fish from the refrigerator and uncover it. Add the cucumbers, tomatoes, onion, and cilantro to the cured fish. Add the set-aside mixture, and combine all ingredients well. Stir in salt and add more to taste. Garnish with diced avocado (if desired). Add tamari and coconut aminos to individual servings (if desired).

This is a large recipe and makes about 10 full servings (or more if you are serving it as an appetizer). Consider cutting the recipe in half if you don't want too many leftovers. Fish is best if eaten the same day, but it can be stored in the refrigerator for up to 3 days. If you do this, separate the juice from the fish so that it does not continue to marinate and overcure.

Serves 10. Per serving: approximately 88 calories, 8.5g carbohydrate, 10g protein, 1.5g fat.

Fall-Apart Crock-Pot Roast (L1/L2/L3M)

3 pounds grass-fed rump roast or
chuck roast

3 tablespoons avocado oil

Salt to rub roast, plus ½ teaspoon,
plus additional

Freshly ground black pepper to rub
roast, plus ½ teaspoon, plus
additional

1 medium onion, diced

1 to 2 teaspoons minced fresh garlic

1 to 2 stalks celery, diced

1 tablespoon tomato paste

1 cup red wine

2 to 3 cups beef broth or bone broth

4 to 8 carrots and/or parsnips,
roughly chopped

4 small red or Yukon Gold potatoes,
roughly chopped

2 cups sliced mushrooms

2 cups fresh or frozen green beans

3 sprigs fresh thyme or more to taste

3 sprigs fresh rosemary or more to
taste

Place a large skillet over medium-high heat. Rub the whole roast with 2 tablespoons of the oil. Salt and pepper both sides of the roast, and then sear it in the skillet until it is a caramelized brown. Remove the roast from the pan, and place it in a Crock-Pot.

In the same skillet, add another tablespoon of the oil. Also add the onion, garlic, celery, ½ teaspoon salt, and ½ teaspoon pepper. Sauté on medium-high heat until vegetables are tender. Mix in the tomato paste, and let that cook for about a minute. Deglaze the pan by pouring in the wine and broth, heat through, and scrape off all the browned bits on the bottom of the pan. Pour over the roast in the Crock-Pot.

Layer carrots, parsnips, potatoes, mushrooms, green beans, thyme, and rosemary on top of the roast. Salt and pepper to taste.

Put the lid on the Crock-Pot and cook for 6 to 8 hours on low until the meat gets very tender. Move the veggies to the bottom of the Crock-Pot for the last hour of cooking to absorb flavor and juices.

Once again, add salt and pepper to taste.

This is a complete meal in one pot.

Modification: L3—Substitute wine with broth.

Serves 8. Per serving: approximately 578 calories, 19.5 carbohydrate, 33g protein, 39g fat (without wine).

Italian Nut Crumbs Meatballs (L1)

Recipe adapted from Susan Laughlin, founder of Nut Crumbs (NutCrumbs.com)

1 pound ground turkey

1 pound grass-fed ground beef or lamb

1 large egg, plus 2 more

½ cup, plus ½ cup Italian Nut Crumbs

½ cup grated Parmesan cheese

Salt and freshly ground black pepper (optional)

1 small onion, chopped (optional)

¼ cup unsweetened almond or coconut milk

¼ cup avocado oil

2 tablespoons ghee

1 (25-ounce) jar marinara sauce

In a large bowl, thoroughly combine the ground meat, 1 egg, ½ cup Nut Crumbs, and cheese. Add salt and pepper (if desired), but the Italian Nut Crumbs have so much flavor and seasoning that this is optional. Add onion (if desired).

In a small bowl, whisk together the remaining 2 eggs and milk.

Pour the remaining ½ cup Nut Crumbs onto a plate.

Form meatballs into 2-inch rounds to ensure the ground turkey will be fully cooked in the middle. Dunk the meatballs in the egg mixture, and then roll them in the Nut Crumbs.

In a skillet, add the oil and ghee and heat them on medium-high. Once the pan is hot, add the meatballs. Cook them for about 2 minutes on one side, and then rotate them. Flip the meatballs every 2 minutes until all sides of them are browned. Add the marinara sauce, cover the skillet, reduce heat to medium-low, and simmer for another hour or until cooked through.

Serving Suggestion: Pour over spaghetti squash or zucchini noodles.

Serves 10. Per serving: approximately 356 calories, 7.5g carbohydrate, 21g protein, 27g fat.

Slow-Cook Chili (L1/L2M/L3M)

2 (16-ounce) cans kidney beans,
   rinsed and drained
1 (16-ounce) can white beans, rinsed
   and drained
1 (16-ounce) can black beans, rinsed
   and drained
1 pound grass-fed ground beef or
   ground turkey, browned and
   crumbled
1 (16-ounce) can stewed tomatoes
1 medium white or yellow onion,
   finely chopped
1 to 2 teaspoons minced fresh garlic
1 to 2 teaspoons cumin and/or chili
   powder
1 (6-ounce) can tomato paste
Dried herbs such as cilantro or
   herbes de Provence (optional)
Salt and freshly ground black pepper

In a Crock-Pot on high setting, place all beans, cooked meat, stewed tomatoes, onion, and garlic. Stir well. Add 1 teaspoon of cumin and/or chili powder at first, and then taste, adding more if you prefer a stronger flavor. Add dried herbs (if desired). Simmer on high for at least 1 hour, and then turn to medium setting for up to 3 hours. Turn Crock-Pot to low until you serve the meal.

Optional Garnishes: Red pepper flakes, grated sharp cheddar, chopped scallions

Time-Saving Tip: Use 4 precooked frozen and thawed Angus patties, crumbled.

Modification: L2/L3—Use diced carrots as a substitute for beans.

Serves 8. Per serving: approximately 290 calories, 61g carbohydrate, 21g protein, 10g fat (beans Level 1 & Lifestyle Phase only).

Sides, Soups, and Sauces

Cauliflower Rice (L1/L2/L3)

1 head cauliflower
1 tablespoon organic extra-virgin
   coconut oil
1 clove garlic, minced
½ cup medium yellow onion,
   chopped
1 teaspoon salt
1 teaspoon freshly ground black
   pepper

Rinse cauliflower under cool water and pat it dry. Using a cheese grater, grate the cauliflower to a coarse texture, approximately the size of rice grains. Or use a food processor to pulse the cauliflower to the desired texture.

In a skillet over medium heat, melt the oil. Sauté the garlic and onion for 3 to 4 minutes, until the onion is relatively translucent. Add in the cauliflower and continue to sauté for 6 to 7 minutes. Season with salt and pepper.

Options: If serving with Mexican-style food, stir in fresh chopped cilantro and a little lime juice. Also delicious covered with our Rich Mushroom Gravy (page 228).

Time-Saving Tip: Precook shredded cauliflower in the microwave for 5 minutes before adding it to the pan.

Serves 4. Per serving: approximately 88 calories, 12.5g carbohydrate, 4.5g protein, 4g fat.

Cauliflower Mash (L1/L2/L3)

1 head cauliflower
2 tablespoons ghee
1 to 2 cloves garlic, minced (optional)
Sea salt
1 to 2 tablespoons canned full-fat
  coconut milk
Chicken or vegetable broth (optional,
  to thin mash if needed)

Cut the cauliflower in half and remove the stem. Chop it into small pieces, and then steam, boil, or cook it until it's tender. Drain the cauliflower in a colander for at least 5 minutes. Place it in a food processor, and pulse it a few times. Add the ghee, the garlic (if desired), and a pinch of sea salt. Pulse again until it's smooth. Add the milk and broth until you get the desired consistency. (You may not need broth if you had a lot of water still in the cauliflower after draining it.) Delicious with Rich Mushroom Gravy (page 228).

Serves 4. Per serving: approximately 126 calories, 11.5g carbohydrate, 4g protein, 8.5g fat.

Sweet Potato Latkes (L1/L2/L3)

3 large eggs, beaten
2 teaspoons coconut flour
¼ teaspoon salt or more to taste
¼ teaspoon garlic powder
¼ teaspoon rosemary or thyme, fresh
  or dried
2 cups shredded yellow sweet potato
  or yam
½ cup finely chopped onion or shallot
2 tablespoons extra-virgin coconut oil

In a medium bowl, mix together the eggs, flour, salt, garlic powder, and rosemary or thyme. Add the potatoes and onion and combine well.

In a large nonstick skillet, melt 1 tablespoon of the oil over medium-low heat. Spoon the potato mixture into the skillet, making 4- to 6-inch pancakes. Cook the first sides for 2 to 3 minutes, until they're golden brown. Flip them and cook another 2 to 3 minutes. Add the second tablespoon of oil to the pan and repeat the cooking method above and complete cooking the entire mixture.

These make a delicious side dish and are great for breakfast too.

Serves 4. Per serving: approximately 215 calories, 25g carbohydrate, 6g protein, 11g fat.

Spicy Nut Crumbs Buffalo Cauliflower (L1)

Recipe adapted from Susan Laughlin, founder of Nut Crumbs (NutCrumbs.com)

2 large eggs, beaten

¼ cup unsweetened almond milk,
    from carton

¼ cup or more Frank's RedHot
    Buffalo Wing Sauce

1 large head cauliflower, chopped into
    florets

½ cup Spicy Nut Crumbs

2 tablespoons avocado oil

In a large bowl, add the eggs and milk and ¼ cup of Frank's RedHot sauce or as much as you'd like. Whisk until the mixture is fully combined. Throw in the cauliflower florets, and make sure they are drenched in the liquid gold.

Pour out the Spicy Nut Crumbs onto a plate, and then dredge the cauliflower in the crumbs until they are fully coated.

Place a medium saucepan on the stove at medium-high heat. Add the oil. When oil is hot, add the cauliflower. Cook it on one side for about 2 minutes, and then use metal tongs to flip it. Cook the other side. Be gentle with the cauliflower and only flip it once so the breading is less likely to fall off.

Once the cauliflower is fully browned, serve it with your favorite dipping sauce. Creamy Ranch Dressing (page 199) would be perfect to serve with these!

Serves 4. Per serving: approximately 198 calories, 10g carbohydrate, 7g protein, 15g fat.

Savory Zucchini Carrot Pancakes (L1/L2/L3)

3 large eggs

2 tablespoons coconut flour (plus additional if needed for a thicker batter)

Sea salt and freshly ground black pepper to taste

1 cup shredded zucchini (hand shred this for quick cleanup—lightly squeeze excess moisture out of shredded zucchini with cheese cloth)

1 cup shredded carrots

2 to 3 scallions, white and green parts, chopped

Dash of garlic powder and/or onion powder (optional)

1 tablespoon extra-virgin coconut oil

Whisk eggs with coconut flour, salt, and pepper. Mix in the zucchini, carrots, scallions, and garlic and/or onion powder (if desired) until combined. Add in additional coconut flour if needed, 1 teaspoon at a time, if the batter seems too thin.

In a medium skillet, heat half the oil over medium heat. Spoon the zucchini batter in to make 4-inch pancakes. Cook them until they're golden brown on bottom, and then flip them once and heat until they're golden brown on the second side before removing from pan. Add rest of oil to pan and repeat with the balance of the mixture. Serve warm.

These make a great side dish but are also good on their own for a savory breakfast or lunch.

Time-Saving Tip: Make a double batch and refrigerate it to reheat for another meal.

Serves 2. Per serving: approximately 182 calories, 9g carbohydrate, 10.5g protein, 11.5g fat.

Quick Roasted Veggies (L1/L2/L3)

4 multicolor carrots, chopped
   (blanched, if desired)
1 cup chopped brussels sprouts
   (blanched, if desired)
1 medium yellow onion, chopped
2 bell peppers (any color), chopped
2 tablespoons extra-virgin coconut
   oil, melted
Herbes de Provence (or any other
   herbs you love)
Sea salt and freshly ground black
   pepper

Optional Glaze
⅛ cup balsamic vinegar
2 teaspoons raw honey

If you want firm veggies, such as carrots or brussels sprouts, to cook more quickly, you can blanch them for about 3 minutes in boiling water and then drain them.

Preheat the oven to 425°F.

In a large ziplock baggie, shake the carrots, brussels sprouts, onion, peppers, and oil. Spread the vegetables one layer deep on a cookie sheet. Sprinkle them with herbs, salt, and pepper. Roast vegetables in the oven for 10 minutes, and then reduce the heat to 350°F and bake for another 10 to 15 minutes.

For the optional glaze, in a small bowl mix together the vinegar and honey. Drizzle over veggies during the last 10 minutes of cooking.

Note: Use any "roast-able" veggie you have on hand, including asparagus, mushrooms, zucchini, squash, eggplant, and broccoli.

Serves 4. Per serving: approximately 125 calories, 15g carbohydrate, 3g protein, 7.5g fat.

Brazilian Cheese Rolls (L1)

¼ cup butter
2 ½ tablespoons unsweetened coconut or almond milk, from carton
2 ½ tablespoons water
½ teaspoon salt
1 cup tapioca flour
1 teaspoon minced fresh garlic
⅓ cup grated or shredded Parmesan cheese
1 large egg, beaten

Preheat the oven to 375°F.

In a small saucepan over high heat, add butter, milk, water, and salt. Bring it to a boil, and then immediately remove it from the heat. Stir in flour and garlic, and continue stirring until mixture is smooth. Set aside the mixture for 10 to 15 minutes.

Stir the cheese and egg into the mixture, and then combine thoroughly until it has a texture similar to that of cottage cheese. Fill a ¼-cup measuring cup approximately three-quarters full and drop rounded mounds of mixture onto an ungreased cookie sheet. Recipe should make 8 medium rolls.

Bake rolls for 15 to 20 minutes or until they're lightly browned on top.

Serves 8. Per serving: approximately 129 calories, 16g carbohydrate, 3g protein, 6g fat.

Roasted Chicken Bone Broth (L1/L2/L3)

1 leftover roasted chicken carcass (cleaned of usable meat)
Vegetable scraps (celery leaves, onion trimmings, carrot peels, garlic)
2 bay leaves
1 tablespoon apple cider vinegar

Place the chicken carcass in a Crock-Pot with vegetable scraps and bay leaves. Pour filtered water to cover and add vinegar. Cook on low heat for 24 hours or longer. Add water as needed. Cook until bones crumble when smashed with a spoon.

Strain the broth through a fine mesh sieve into a freezer-quality container. The broth may gel, but not always. Bone broth can be stored in the refrigerator for no more than a week, or the freezer for up to six months. You can also freeze it in ice cube trays and transfer the frozen cubes of broth to a resealable ziplock freezer bag.

Servings vary. Per serving: 30–60 calories (varies based on amount of water and how much it reduces).

Grain-Free and Delicious Flatbread (L1)

½ cup blanched almond flour
½ cup tapioca flour
1 cup canned full-fat coconut milk
½ teaspoon salt
Optional, if not using nonstick pan: 1
    teaspoon extra-virgin coconut oil,
    avocado oil, or butter (use only for
    greasing pan)

Mix all ingredients in a bowl.

Place a nonstick pan or skillet over no more than medium heat as the flatbread needs to cook somewhat slowly to both brown outside and cook fully inside.

Pour about ¼ cup batter into the skillet. The batter is quite thick, so spread it out a bit with a spatula to create a thin pancake. Cook for 2 minutes until the upper side is fully bubbled across the entire surface and the bottom is starting to brown. Flip and cook the other side for 2 minutes, until it is starting to brown as well. To get a nice crispness, cook each side an additional 1 minute. This specific cooking technique is needed for the flatbread to cook properly inside and out. (If by chance your flatbread comes out slightly gooey inside, place it on an ungreased cookie sheet and bake for 5 to 10 minutes at 350°F.)

Variations: Mix some herbs and/or garlic in the batter. Top the flatbread with ghee or goat cheese. These flatbreads can also be used as a base for mini pizzas—just add toppings and stick the flatbread under the broiler. Or use flatbread as wraps or taco shells. Flatbread is most tasty when it's warm, but you can refrigerate it and then reheat it in your skillet or pan.

Note: This bread is grain free and wheat free but not carbohydrate or calorie free, so eat it in moderation!

Serves 6. Per serving: approximately 156 calories, 12g carbohydrate, 2g protein, 11g fat.

Chicken Vegetable Soup (L1/L2/L3)

1 large onion, chopped
2 cups your choice of veggies (carrots, broccoli, riced or whole cauliflower)
1 cup leftover chopped roasted chicken
5 cups bone broth or organic chicken broth
Herbes de Provence
Salt and freshly ground black pepper

Combine onion, veggies, chicken, broth, herbs, and salt and pepper (to taste) in a saucepan, and heat it until the vegetables are desired tenderness. Simple!

Special Tip: No cooked chicken on hand? Place chicken (frozen or thawed) in a 3-quart soup pan. Pour in 8 cups filtered water and add 2 teaspoons sea salt. Bring to a low boil, and cover until the chicken is mostly cooked (10 to 12 minutes). Remove from the heat, and chop the chicken into small pieces. Add to broth and veggies.

Serves 8. Per serving: approximately 65 calories, 4g carbohydrate, 5g protein, 1g fat (serving size: 1 cup).

Kale Potato Soup (L1/L2/L3)

1 ½ quarts organic chicken or bone broth
1 pound spicy chicken sausage (or any meat you choose)
1 tablespoon extra-virgin coconut oil
1 cup chopped onion
1 to 1 ½ cups chopped celery
1 large sweet potato, peeled and diced
4 to 5 cups fresh or packaged chopped kale
Sea salt and freshly ground black pepper
Dried parsley, herbes de Provence, or other spices of your choice
¼ to ½ cup canned full-fat coconut milk

In a medium saucepan over medium-high heat, bring the broth to a boil.

Meanwhile, in a large skillet over medium-high heat, brown the meat. Add the oil, onion, and celery. Sauté until celery is cooked and onion is golden brown. Remove from heat.

Once the broth is at a boil, transfer the meat, celery, and onion to the broth. Add the potatoes and continue cooking until they are very soft. Add kale and cook until it is soft and shrunken, followed by the salt, pepper, and your favorite spices. Slowly stir in ¼ to ½ cup of the milk, according to your creaminess preference.

Serves 8. Per serving: approximately 64 calories, 4g carbohydrate, 4g protein, 5g fat.

Carrot Ginger Soup (L1/L2/L3)

2 teaspoons extra-virgin coconut oil
1 tablespoon minced fresh ginger
1 tablespoon minced shallot
4 cups thinly sliced carrots
3 cups chicken or vegetable broth
Sea salt and freshly ground black
    pepper
¼ cup canned full-fat coconut milk
    (optional)

Place oil in a large saucepan over medium-low heat. When oil is hot, add the ginger and shallot and sauté until soft, about 3 to 5 minutes. Add the carrots and sauté until caramelized and tender, about 12 to 15 minutes. Add the broth and cook until all veggies are very tender, about 10 more minutes. Sprinkle with a little salt. Remove from heat and transfer to a blender.

Puree or blend to desired consistency. (If using a regular blender, be sure to do this in batches and cover the lid with a towel so the blender does not overflow.) If you like a creamy soup, return the mixture to the saucepan and add the milk. Add salt and pepper to taste. If you prefer soup extra warm, reheat in original saucepan for 1 to 2 minutes on medium heat.

Serves 4. Per serving: approximately 142 calories, 15g carbohydrate, 3g protein, 9g fat.

Red Curry Pumpkin Soup (L1/L2/L3)

2 to 4 tablespoons Thai Kitchen Red
    Curry Paste
2 (15-ounce) cans pumpkin puree
Salt
4 cups chicken broth or any flavor
    bone broth
1 can full-fat coconut milk
¼ teaspoon dried ginger (optional)
⅛ teaspoon cayenne pepper
    (optional)
Red pepper flakes (optional)
Freshly ground black pepper
    (optional)
Cinnamon (optional)
Drizzle of raw honey (optional)

Add Red Curry Paste to a soup pot over medium heat. Cook for 1 to 2 minutes, until fragrant.

Add pumpkin, salt, and broth. Stir and cook for approximately 3 minutes until it's lightly bubbling. Stir in the milk and cook another 3 to 4 minutes. Add ginger and cayenne pepper at this time to taste (if desired). To garnish, sprinkle with red pepper flakes, ground black pepper, or cinnamon, or drizzle with raw honey.

Serves 8. Per serving: approximately 125 calories, 11g carbohydrate, 5g protein, 10g fat, 4g fiber.

10-Minute Asparagus Soup (L1/L2/L3)

8 asparagus stalks, trimmed
⅓ cup chopped shallot or onion
    (optional)
Chicken or vegetable broth (enough
    to cover veggies in pot)
¼ teaspoon salt
¼ teaspoon freshly ground black
    pepper
½ teaspoon herbes de Provence

Add asparagus and shallot or onion (if desired) to soup pot. Pour in enough broth to just cover vegetables. Add seasonings. You may need to add more broth as vegetables cook. Keep pot on medium-high heat until the broth is bubbling and vegetables are tender. Allow to cool just a bit, and then transfer to a blender. Blend until smooth. Add salt and pepper. Enjoy!

Variations for Soup:

Celery
Broccoli
Carrots
Bell peppers
Canned coconut milk for creamier version
Curry

Serves 2. Per serving: approximately 42 calories, 7g carbohydrate, 2g protein, 2.5g fat (serving size: approximately 1 cup).

Rich Mushroom Gravy (L1/L2/L3)

2 tablespoons organic butter or ghee
1 small onion, finely chopped
1 ½ cups finely chopped mushrooms
3 to 4 teaspoons arrowroot
2 cups vegetable broth
Salt and freshly ground black pepper

Melt the butter in a saucepan over medium heat. Add the onion and sauté until it's dark golden-brown. Add the mushrooms and cook for an additional 2 minutes. Stir in 3 teaspoons arrowroot. Cook gently for 1 minute, and then gradually add vegetable broth. Bring to a boil, stirring constantly, until thickened and blended. Remove from heat, and add salt and pepper to taste.

Tip: If the sauce is not thick enough, add 1 additional teaspoon of arrowroot at a time using the following method: Take 1 teaspoon arrowroot, add 1 teaspoon water, stir until dissolved, and then add it to your gravy and stir. Bring to a boil again while stirring. The gravy should thicken to the desired consistency.

Serves 8. Per serving: approximately 40 calories, 3g carbohydrate, 1g protein, 3g fat (serving size: ¼ cup).

Fresh Pesto (L1/L2M/L3M)

2 cups packed fresh basil leaves
(substitutions: arugula, kale)
¼ cup raw or toasted nuts, such as
walnuts, pine nuts, or pecans
3 garlic cloves, minced
½ cup grated pecorino or Parmesan
cheese
½ cup extra-virgin olive oil
Salt and freshly ground black pepper

Combine the basil leaves and nuts in a food processor, and pulse several times. Add the garlic and cheese, and pulse several times more. Scrape down the sides of the processor with a rubber spatula, and on low speed slowly add the oil. Occasionally stop to scrape down sides. Add salt and pepper to taste, and then pulse again several times.

Using a blender or a bullet, place all ingredients in at once and blend for 15-second intervals until blended. Add salt and pepper to taste. Blend one more time.

Serve on vegetables, spaghetti squash, zoodles (zucchini noodles), fish, and more!

Modifications: L2/L3—Make the pesto without cheese and substitute pumpkin seeds or sunflower seeds for nuts. You may also delete any nut or seed and make with just basil, garlic, and oil.

Makes approximately 16 tablespoons. Per tablespoon: approximately 87 calories, less than 1g carbohydrate, less than 1g protein, 9g fat.

Desserts and Treats

Fast and Creamy Berry Sorbet (L1/L2/L3)

1 cup berries (fresh or frozen)
2 ripe bananas (preferably overripe, fresh or frozen)
¼ cup canned full-fat coconut milk

In a blender or bullet, blend until smooth. Freeze until it's the consistency you like.

Serves 4. Per serving: approximately 100 calories, 18g carbohydrate, 10g sugar, 3g fat, 3g fiber.

Berry Compote Cake (L1/L2/L3)

1 tablespoon, plus ¼ cup extra-virgin coconut oil, melted
4 cups frozen or fresh mixed berries (thaw and drain if using frozen)
½ lemon, juiced
Zest of ½ lemon
⅛ teaspoon pure monk fruit extract or sweetener of your preference to taste
4 large eggs
¼ cup raw honey or pure maple syrup
½ cup unsweetened coconut or almond milk
2 teaspoons pure vanilla extract
½ cup coconut flour
¼ teaspoon cinnamon
1 teaspoon baking soda
¼ teaspoon salt

Preheat the oven to 400°F.

In an 8 x 8 x 2-inch baking dish, add 1 tablespoon of the oil, berries, lemon juice, and lemon zest. If desired, add a natural sweetener of choice to the berries.

In a medium bowl, mix together the eggs, ¼ cup of the oil, honey or syrup, milk, and vanilla. Mix in the flour, cinnamon, baking soda, and salt until a batter is formed. If desired, add sweetener to taste. Drop the batter by spoonful over the top of the fruit and smooth over the top. It does not need to completely cover the berry mixture because it will spread out as it bakes.

Bake the cake for 10 minutes, and then reduce the oven to 375°F and continue to bake it for 30 to 40 minutes or until the fruit is bubbly and the top is golden brown. Let cool for a few minutes. This cake is best served warm, but it is delicious cold as well.

Serves 8. Per serving: approximately 207 calories, 20g carbohydrate, 13g sugar, 4g protein, 11g fat (1 serving counts as ½ tablespoon honey or syrup).

Sun Cookies (L1M/L2/L3)

6 tablespoons raw honey or pure maple syrup

1 large egg, beaten

½ teaspoon salt

½ teaspoon baking soda

⅛ teaspoon pure monk fruit extract or sweetener of your preference to taste

1 cup unsweetened sunflower seed butter (such as SunButter)

Preheat the oven to 375°F.

In a medium bowl, stir together the honey or syrup, egg, salt, baking soda, and sweetener. Stir well. Add the butter and mix until the batter is fully combined and starting to thicken. If you want to increase sweetness, add stevia or lo han to taste.

Dollop about 1 tablespoon batter per cookie onto a parchment-covered cookie sheet. Bake cookies for 15 to 20 minutes until they're golden brown. Slide parchment paper off the pan and allow the cookies to cool.

Modification: L1/LS—If you are not sensitive to peanuts, you can substitute organic Valencia peanut butter in place of seed butter.

Makes 18 cookies. Per cookie: approximately 113 calories, 6g carbohydrate, 4.5g sugar, 4g protein, 7.5g fat (1 cookie counts as 1 teaspoon honey/maple syrup).

Dark Chocolate Truffles (L1/L2/L3)

½ cup extra-virgin coconut oil

½ cup coconut butter (coconut manna)

¾ cup cocoa powder

¼ cup raw honey or pure maple syrup

1 teaspoon pure vanilla extract

¼ teaspoon salt

1/16 to ⅛ teaspoon pure monk fruit extract or sweetener of your preference to taste

½ cup chopped almonds or peanuts (optional)

Coarse sea salt (optional)

In a small saucepan over low heat, melt oil and butter. Stir until blended. Add cocoa and mix until combined and it looks like a liquid chocolate sauce. Turn off the heat. Mix in honey or syrup, vanilla, and salt. Add sweetener and nuts (if desired). Stir until mixture is evenly combined.

Pour the mixture into silicone candy molds, and then put the molds in the freezer until the chocolate sets solid. If you don't have silicone molds, use plastic ice cube trays and fill them about half full. If desired, sprinkle with coarse sea salt to taste.

Makes 38 pieces. Per piece: approximately 63 calories, 4g carbohydrate, 2.5g sugar, 5g fat (without nuts).

Chocolate Coconut Macaroons (L1/L2/L3)

3 cups shredded unsweetened coconut
½ cup cocoa powder
½ cup raw honey or pure maple syrup
½ cup canned full-fat coconut milk
½ teaspoon cinnamon
⅛ teaspoon pure monk fruit extract or sweetener of your preference to taste
¼ teaspoon pure vanilla extract
1 large egg white
Pinch of sea salt

Preheat the oven to 325°F.

In a large bowl, combine coconut, cocoa, honey or syrup, milk, cinnamon, sweetener, and vanilla. Stir thoroughly. In a small mixing bowl, use a mixer to beat the egg white and salt for about 2 minutes, or until fluffy peaks are formed.

Fold egg-white mixture into chocolate mixture and gently combine. Scoop balls of the mixture using a tablespoon and pack down firmly onto a cookie sheet lined with parchment paper. Bake for 30 minutes. Let cool and enjoy.

Makes about 22 macaroons. Per macaroon: approximately 100 calories, 10g carbohydrate, 4g sugar, 8g fat, 2g fiber (1 macaroon counts as 1 teaspoon honey/maple syrup).

Chocolate Bliss Squares (L1/L2/L3)

1 cup extra-virgin coconut oil (warmed to liquid state)
¼ cup raw honey or pure maple syrup
2 teaspoons pure vanilla extract
⅛ teaspoon pure monk fruit extract or sweetener of your preference to taste
¼ teaspoon sea salt
1 cup dried shredded unsweetened coconut
¾ to 1 cup cocoa powder

Using a mixer or blender or by hand, blend the oil, honey or syrup, vanilla, sweetener, and salt. Add the coconut (½ cup at a time), and blend until smooth. Stir in the cocoa until the ingredients are thoroughly combined. Adjust your amount of cocoa so that your batter is the consistency of brownie batter.

Line the bottom of an 8 x 8 x 2-inch baking pan with parchment paper. Pour in the mixture. Place it in the refrigerator or freezer until it's solid. Once the mixture is solid, the parchment paper will peel away easily and the chocolate can be cut into squares. Store all finished squares in the refrigerator or freezer to prevent melting.

Makes 20 1-ounce pieces. Per piece: approximately 160 calories, 7g carbohydrate, 4.5g sugar, 14g fat (1 piece counts as ¼ tablespoon honey or syrup).

Energy Bites (L1/L2M/L3M)

½ cup almond butter

⅛ cup raw honey

½ cup shredded unsweetened coconut, plus extra for coating

1 tablespoon chia seeds

½ cup chopped pumpkin or sun-flower seeds

⅛ teaspoon sea salt

⅛ cup cocoa powder (optional, for rolling)

1/16 to ⅛ teaspoon pure monk fruit extract or sweetener of your preference to taste

In a medium bowl, add the butter, honey, coconut, chia seeds, pumpkin or sunflower seeds, and salt. Mix well. Form rounded tablespoons of the mixture into balls, and then roll them in a little shredded coconut or cocoa powder and refrigerate.

Modification: L2/L3—Substitute unsweetened sunflower butter for almond butter.

Makes 16 bites. Per bite: approximately 100 calories, 5g carbohydrate, 3g sugar, 3g protein, 8g fat.

Banana Mug Cake (L1/L2/L3)

2 large ripe bananas, mashed well (the browner the better!)

1 large egg, lightly beaten

2 tablespoons canned full-fat coco-nut milk (unsweetened)

4 tablespoons coconut flour

½ teaspoon cinnamon

½ teaspoon baking soda

Pinch of sea salt

1/16 teaspoon pure monk fruit extract or sweetener of your preference to taste (optional)

Mix the bananas, egg, and milk together in a me-dium bowl. In a small bowl, sift or just mix together the flour, cinnamon, baking soda, and salt. Add sweetener (if desired). Add dry ingredients to wet ones, and mix until combined into a batter. Scoop and divide the batter evenly into 2 microwave-safe coffee mugs. Place mugs individually in the micro-wave for 3 minutes each. Allow the cake to cool for 3 to 4 minutes. Enjoy right from the mug, or use a knife to loosen the edges and flip the mugs over to release the cake onto plates.

Serves 2. Per serving: approximately 223 calories, 36g carbohydrate, 6g protein, 7g fat, 8g fiber.

Grain-Free Banana Bread (Lifestyle Phase Only)

¼ cup extra-virgin coconut oil, plus extra for greasing pan

½ cup raw honey or pure maple syrup

2 large eggs

⅛ teaspoon pure monk fruit extract or sweetener of your preference to taste

½ teaspoon pure vanilla extract

1½ cups mashed ripe bananas

1¼ cups cassava flour

½ teaspoon salt

½ cup chopped pecans or walnuts (optional)

Preheat the oven to 375°F.

In a medium bowl, combine the oil, honey or syrup, eggs, sweetener, and vanilla, and stir until it's creamy. Stir in mashed bananas. Add flour, salt, and nuts (if desired) to mixture and combine well.

Grease a 9 x 5 x 3-inch loaf pan with oil. If desired, line the bottom of the loaf pan with parchment paper so the bread slips right out after it is baked. Pour batter into loaf pan. Bake for 45 to 50 minutes, or until the top and sides become golden brown and a toothpick inserted into the center comes out dry.

Serves 10. Per serving: approximately 137 calories, 34g carbohydrate, 18g sugar, 1.5g protein, 6.5g fat (without nuts).

Beverages

Sparkling Cranberry Mocktail (L1/L2/L3)

2 to 4 ounces unsweetened
  cranberry juice
6 to 8 ounces sparkling water
3 to 4 cubes of ice
Liquid stevia or liquid lo han

Pour juice and water over ice in a glass. Sweeten to taste and stir for a refreshing mocktail.

Serves 1. Per serving: approximately 18 calories, 4g carbohydrate, 2.5g sugar.

Sparkling Lemonade (L1/L2/L3)

2 tablespoons fresh lemon juice
6 to 8 ounces sparkling water
3 to 4 cubes of ice
Liquid stevia or liquid lo han

Pour juice and water over ice in a glass. Sweeten to taste, stir, and serve.

Serves 1. Per serving: approximately 10 calories.

A Note from Danna and Robyn

We are honored that you chose to read this book and allowed us to come alongside you on your journey toward a leaner and healthier body. It is our hope and prayer that you found lasting solutions that will serve you well for a lifetime. We'd love to continue supporting you in moving toward your goals and invite you to join us in community with other women through the free resources shared on the next page.

We'd be delighted to hear from you and learn how your lifestyle is changing. You can email us directly at Support@EatLiveThriveDiet.com.

We sincerely believe that your best years are ahead of you.

God's richest blessings,
Danna and Robyn

Resources for Your Journey

A Website Dedicated to Supporting Your Journey

We've created a free website to help you on your journey to turn back the scale and the clock. There are several helpful worksheets and logs that you can download as needed, as well as additional tools and resources to enhance your experience. Simply go to EatLiveThriveDiet.com and register with your email address to obtain unlimited access.

LeanHealthyAgeless.com—A Free Resource for Women

We love encouraging women of all ages in their health, weight loss, and life journey. We post blogs, videos, cooking shows, and other resources every month. Please join us at LeanHealthy Ageless.com.

Lean Healthy Ageless Facebook Page

We invite you to engage with us and a community of like-minded women on Facebook. We post regularly and answer many of your questions.

Eat Live Thrive Academy Membership

For a small monthly fee, you can have access to an exclusive membership for women that includes weekly live health and weight-loss coaching and extensive health, nutrition, and weight-loss resources and support. The academy is designed to encourage, educate, and equip women to deal with the challenges of aging and live life to the fullest. For more information, visit EatLiveThrive Academy.com.

Healthy Self-Talk CDs and MP3s

The following titles can be found on our web store at LeanHealthyAgeless.com.

- *Eat, Live, Thrive Diet Self-Talk*
- *Change Your Habits...By Renewing Your Mind!*
- *Healthy Self-Talk for Your Lifestyle*
- *Self-Talk for a Contented Life*

Acknowledgments

First and foremost, we want to thank our Lord and Savior, Jesus, for the inspiration and motivation to write this book. It started as an outflow from a podcast about a gentle cleansing/detox regime. From there, it morphed into a complete diet and lifestyle plan as the women we coached realized fantastic results.

In the ever-changing world of nutrition, it is challenging to discern fact from fiction, and positive trends from passing fads. A registered dietician with a master's and PhD as well as other specialty certifications too numerous to name, Patti Milligan has been a generous friend and consultant to us throughout the journey of writing this book. Her broad scope of knowledge and balanced approach to nutrition helped us ensure that our diet recommendations and philosophies were sound. Plus, Patti has a unique approach that causes people to celebrate nutritious food without sacrificing a fully satisfying taste-bud celebration.

Mark Stengler, NMD, is a brilliant practitioner who stays on top of the most reliable studies and best practices in natural medicine. We are thankful for his willingness to be available at a moment's notice to provide accurate and credible science to support many references in this book. We also appreciate how he has graciously educated us over the years in our own health journeys. His wise guidance has given us confidence to continue to pursue health in the most natural ways possible. It is a breath of fresh air to have a doctor who is willing to listen to our countless questions and comments about the female body, hormones, and aging with great understanding and a sense of humor when needed. We are blessed to have him as our personal doctor, adviser, and friend.

Our sincere thanks to Victoria Bowmann, PhD, for spending time with us on the phone and in video-chat sessions to answer many questions about the complexity of the digestive system. It is a topic that many people aren't always comfortable discussing. Victoria makes it easy to ask very direct, descriptive questions without embarrassment and provides clear and easy-to-understand and sometimes humorous answers. Her knowledge and approach made it easy for us to not only "digest" complex topics and write about them in a way that women can understand but also appreciate why these issues are so essential to total health.

We all need mentors and experts who not only encourage us but also tell us the truth. We love that our agent, Steve Laube, tells it like it is. If an idea is great, he is all over it. If it's not, he is the first to give us a kind (and often humorous) reality check. We are also thankful that he is so well respected in the industry that relative unknowns such as us can get our best ideas in front of great publishers. We are already looking forward to our next project with you, Steve!

We are so jazzed that God gave us the ultimate publishing dream team. We are grateful that Laura Barker saw something intriguing in our book and knew that Susan Tjaden would be a fantastic fit as our senior editor. We personally clicked from our first conversation and have been blown away by her enthusiasm and support throughout our journey. As she introduced us to other dynamic "ageless" women who shared her enthusiasm at WaterBrook—Ginia Hairston Croker, Lisa Beech, and Ingrid Beck—we realized that we could not have hand selected a more perfect group of women to champion this project. A thank-you also to Anita Palmer for her insightful edits and revisions. Helen Macdonald, we appreciated your grace and patience guiding us through the final typesetting and edits on our tight deadline. And a special thanks to Tina Constable, who nudged us to keep working until we found just the right title to describe the true experience and result we hope women will enjoy.

Last and certainly not least, we want to thank our husbands (Lew Boore and Rob Thomson) for their unwavering support of our commitment to encouraging women in their quests for healthier bodies and more balanced lifestyles. We realize that our tight deadline on this book cut into a lot of our personal family time. Your patience and belief in us mean more than you can know.

And to you, our reader, we truly do want you to eat, live, and thrive in ways that ensure you realize your best body and health, no matter your age!

Notes

Chapter 1: Yes, You Can Eat, Live, and Thrive!

1. Yurdagül Zopf, MD, et al., "The Differential Diagnosis of Food Intolerance," *Deutsches Ärzteblatt International* 106, no. 21 (May 2009): 359–70, www.ncbi.nlm.nih.gov/pmc/articles/PMC2695393.

2. "Lactose Intolerance," Genetics Home Reference, May 2010, https://ghr.nlm.nih.gov/condition/lactose-intolerance#definition.

3. Ron Milo, PhD, and Rob Phillips, PhD, "How Quickly Do Different Cells in the Body Replace Themselves?," Cell Biology by the Numbers, http://book.bionumbers.org/how-quickly-do-different-cells-in-the-body-replace-themselves.

4. Patti Milligan, RD, MS, PhD, in discussion with the authors, May 2018.

5. Robert Lustig, MD, interview by Dr. Joseph Mercola, "Research Proves Causation—Sugar Consumption Increases Risk for Chronic Disease," Mercola, January 25, 2015, https://articles.mercola.com/sites/articles/archive/2015/01/25/sugar-increases-chronic-disease-risk.aspx.

6. Andreas Eenfeldt, MD, "Professor Lustig: 'Insulin Drives All of the Behaviors Seen in Obesity,'" *Diet Doctor* (blog), April 24, 2017, www.dietdoctor.com/professor-lustig-insulin-drives-behaviours-seen-obesity.

Chapter 2: Making the Program Work for You

1. This is the motto for the Dr. Axe website. See Jillian Levy, CHHC, "Food Is Medicine: The Diet of Medicinal Foods, Science and History," Dr. Axe, June 13, 2016, https://draxe.com/food-is-medicine.

Chapter 3: You Are What You Think

1. Alia Crum, quoted in Alix Spiegel, "Mind over Milkshake: How Your Thoughts Fool Your Stomach," NPR Morning Edition, April 14, 2014, www.npr.org/sections/health-shots/2014/04/14/299179468/mind-over-milkshake-how-your-thoughts-fool-your-stomach.

2. Bob George, *Classic Christianity: Life's Too Short to Miss the Real Thing* (Eugene, OR: Harvest House, 1989), 9.

3. Signe Dean, "Here's How Long It Really Takes to Break a Habit, According to Science," Science Alert, June 9, 2018, www.sciencealert.com/how-long-it-takes-to-break-a-habit-according-to-science.

Chapter 4: The Power of Self-Talk

1. William Backus, PhD, *The Healing Power of a Christian Mind: How Biblical Truth Can Keep You Healthy* (Minneapolis, MN: Bethany, 1996), 9–10, 13, 28, 52.
2. Shad Helmstetter, PhD, "The Story of Self-Talk," video, 7:10, April 30, 2008, www.youtube.com/watch?v=rvzfnm9uk-0.

Chapter 5: Fat-Burning Diet Trends

1. William Cole, DC, IFMCP, "Is Intermittent Fasting Bad for Your Hormones? These Are the Pros and Cons," Mind Body Green, October 17, 2017, www.mindbodygreen.com/articles/is-intermittent-fasting-bad-for-your-hormones-these-are-the-pros-cons.
2. Erica Kannall, "How Does Your Body Store Excess Calories?," SFGate, updated April 3, 2018, https://healthyeating.sfgate.com/body-store-excess-calories-9627.html.
3. "Farm Wife, 1900," EyeWitness to History, 2007, www.eyewitnesstohistory.com/farm wife.htm.
4. Cyrus Khambatta, PhD, "You Are 'When' You Eat," www.mangomannutrition.com/you-are-when-you-eat-intermittent-fasting.
5. Valter D. Longo and Mark P. Mattson, "Fasting: Molecular Mechanisms and Clinical Applications," *Cell Metabolism* 19, no. 2 (February 2014): 181–92, https://doi.org/10.1016/j.cmet.2013.12.008.
6. Mark Stengler, NMD, www.markstengler.com.
7. Catherine R. Marinac et al., "Prolonged Nightly Fasting and Breast Cancer Prognosis," *JAMA Oncology* 2, no. 8 (August 2016): 1049–55, www.ncbi.nlm.nih.gov/pmc/articles/PMC4982776.
8. Dr. Joseph Mercola, "How Intermittent Fasting Stacks Up Among Obesity-Related Myths, Assumptions, and Evidence-Backed Facts," Peak Fitness, March 1, 2013, https://fitness.mercola.com/sites/fitness/archive/2013/03/01/daily-intermittent-fasting.aspx.
9. Michelle Harvie, PhD, and Anthony Howell, FRCP, "Potential Benefits and Harms of Intermittent Energy Restriction and Intermittent Fasting Amongst Obese, Overweight and Normal Weight Subjects—A Narrative Review of Human and Animal Evidence," *Behavioral Sciences* 7, no. 1 (March 2017), www.ncbi.nlm.nih.gov/pmc/articles/PMC5371748.

10. "Ketogenic Diet," Epilepsy Society, March 2016, www.epilepsysociety.org.uk/ketogenic-diet#.W4RG4i3My9Y.

11. Marcelo Campos, MD, "Ketogenic Diet: Is the Ultimate Low-Carb Diet Good for You?" *Harvard Health Blog,* July 27, 2017, www.health.harvard.edu/blog/ketogenic-diet-is-the-ultimate-low-carb-diet-good-for-you-2017072712089.

Chapter 7: The Elimination Phase

1. Eric Troy, "What Is the Origin of the Word Diet?," August 26, 2014, CulinaryLore.com, https://culinarylore.com/food-history:origin-of-the-word-diet.

2. Victoria Bowmann, PhD (homeopathist), May 5, 2018, in discussion with Robyn. More information is available at her website, www.MyRealHealth.com.

3. "How to Use the Glycemic Index," WebMD, reviewed by Michael Dansinger, MD, on January 17, 2017, www.webmd.com/diabetes/guide/glycemic-index-good-versus-bad-carbs#1.

Chapter 8: The Discovery Phase

1. Mark Stengler, NMD, email message to authors.

2. "How Much Is Too Much? The Growing Concern over Too Much Added Sugar in Our Diets," UCSF: SugarScience, http://sugarscience.ucsf.edu/the-growing-concern-of-overconsumption.html#.W4Rc5i3My9Y; see also Kris Gunnars, BSc, "11 Graphs That Show Everything That Is Wrong with the Modern Diet," Healthline, June 8, 2017, www.healthline.com/nutrition/11-graphs-that-show-what-is-wrong-with-modern-diet.

3. Mark Hyman, MD, "Top 10 Big Ideas: How to Detox from Sugar," *Dr. Hyman* (blog), March 6, 2014, http://drhyman.com/blog/2014/03/06/top-10-big-ideas-detox-sugar.

Chapter 9: The Lifestyle Phase

1. Ty Bollinger, "The Sugar and Cancer Connection: Why Sugar Is Called 'The White Death,'" Truth About Cancer, September 2016, www.thetruthaboutcancer.com/sugar-white-death.

Chapter 10: Notched-Up Nutrition

1. Dr. Joseph Mercola, "7 Worst Ingredients in Food," Mercola, December 30, 2013, https://articles.mercola.com/sites/articles/archive/2013/12/30/worst-food-ingredients.aspx.

2. "About Genetically Engineered Foods," Center for Food Safety, www.centerforfoodsafety.org/issues/311/ge-foods/about-ge-foods.

3. Dr. Joseph Mercola, "New Study of Splenda (Sucralose) Reveals Shocking Information About Potential Harmful Effects," Mercola, February 10, 2009, https://articles.mercola.com/sites/articles/archive/2009/02/10/new-study-of-splenda-reveals-shocking-information-about-potential-harmful-effects.aspx.
4. Melis Ann, "The Negative Side Effects of Eating Genetically-Modified Foods," Soapboxie, May 30, 2018, https://soapboxie.com/social-issues/What-Genetically-Modified-Foods-Do-to-Our-Bodies.
5. Andrew Weil, MD, "4 Ways to Avoid Meat with Added Growth Hormones," Weil, www.drweil.com/blog/health-tips/are-you-eating-meat-with-added-growth-hormones.
6. Annie Price, CHHC, "Antibiotics in Fast Food: See How 25 Top Chains Rank," Dr. Axe, October 18, 2016, https://draxe.com/antibiotics-in-fast-food.
7. Rachel Thompson, PhD, "Red Meat and Bowel Cancer Risk—How Strong Is the Evidence?," *World Cancer Research Fund International* (blog), October 23, 2015, www.wcrf.org/int/blog/articles/2015/10/red-meat-and-bowel-cancer-risk-how-strong-evidence.
8. Kissairis Munoz, "Bacon-Gate: Will Eating Red or Processed Meat Cause Cancer?," Dr. Axe, November 6, 2015, https://draxe.com/processed-meat.
9. William D. Lassek, MD, and Steven J. C. Gaulin, PhD, *Why Women Need Fat: How "Healthy" Food Makes Us Gain Excess Weight and the Surprising Solution to Losing It Forever* (New York: Hudson Street, 2012), 31–32.
10. Dr. Joseph Mercola, "Omega-3 Level Is the Best Predictor of Mortality," Mercola, April 2, 2018, https://articles.mercola.com/sites/articles/archive/2018/04/02/omega-3-level-mortality-predictor.aspx.
11. Josh Axe, DC, DNM, "The Risks and Benefits of Drinking Coffee," Dr. Axe, September 22, 2015, https://draxe.com/benefits-of-drinking-coffee.
12. Robert Tornambe, MD, "Fish Oil for Your Face? The New Anti-Aging Phenomenon," *Huffington Post* (blog), December 17, 2011, www.huffingtonpost.com/robert-tornambe-md/omega-3-anti-aging-_b_993047.html.

Chapter 12: What's Exercise Got to Do with It?

1. "Why You're Not Losing Weight: A Q & A with Dr. Sara Gottfried," Goop, https://goop.com/wellness/health/why-youre-not-losing-weight.

Chapter 13: The Irreplaceable Power of Sleep

1. Scott Christ, "The Effect of Sleep on Muscle Growth, According to Science," *Pure Food* (blog), www.purefoodcompany.com/effect-sleep-on-muscle-growth.

2. Sanjay R. Patel, MD, et al., "Association Between Reduced Sleep and Weight Gain in Women," *American Journal of Epidemiology* 164, no. 10 (November 2006): 947–54, www.ncbi.nlm.nih .gov/pmc/articles/PMC3496783.

3. Shahrad Taheri, PhD, et al., "Short Sleep Duration Is Associated with Reduced Leptin, Elevated Ghrelin, and Increased Body Mass Index," *PLOS Medicine* 1, no. 3 (December 2004), http:// journals.plos.org/plosmedicine/article?id=10.1371/journal.pmed.0010062.

4. "Brain Basics: Understanding Sleep," National Institute of Neurological Disorders and Stroke, July 6, 2018, www.ninds.nih.gov/Disorders/Patient-Caregiver-Education/Understanding -Sleep#2. See also Max Hirshkowitz, PhD, et al., "National Sleep Foundation's Sleep Time Duration Recommendations: Methodology and Results Summary," *Sleep Health* 1, no. 1 (March 2015): 40–43, www.sleephealthjournal.org/article/S2352-7218%2815%2900015 -7/fulltext.

Chapter 14: Beauty and the Beast

1. Carolyn Mahaney and Nicole Whitacre, *True Beauty* (Wheaton, IL: Crossway, 2014), 38–39.

Index

A

activity, 54, 72–73, 74
additives, 132
adrenal fatigue, 52, 74, 139
aerobic exercise, 162
affirmation statements, 25
alcoholic beverages, 66, 91,
   139–42, 169
almond milk, 55
Alzheimer's disease, 41, 138
American Journal of Epidemiology,
   168
American restaurant cuisines, 149
anti-aging strategy for skin, 142
antibiotic resistance, 135
antibiotics, 134–38
apple cider vinegar, 68, 126
artificial sweeteners, 114, 133
Atkins, Robert, 43
attitudes
   on beauty, 175–76, 179–80
   habits and, 24, 29–33
   minds, transformation of, 24–26
   spiritual transformation, 26
   thoughts influences, 21–26
   unhealthy thoughts, 30–31
   See also self-talk
autophagy, 41
avocados, 144
Axe, Josh, 17, 135, 139

B

Backus, William, 28
basal metabolic rate (BMR), 81,
   121, 123
BBQ restaurant cuisines, 151
beans (legumes), 95–96

beauty
   the Bible and, 176–78
   perceptions of, 175–76, 179–80
beer, 141
Behavioral Sciences journal, 43
beliefs, impact of, 22
beverages and liquids, 62, 68–69
   See also alcoholic beverages;
     water, drinking
blood sugar, 14, 52
blueberries, 144
body
   brushing, 71, 74
   changes, 12
   response to fasting, 35–36
   stress effects, 160
   See also exercise
bok choy, 144
Bollinger, Ty, 114
bone broth, 55, 75, 143
Boulder Canyon Potato Chips,
   153
bowel movements, 75
Bowmann, Victoria, 75–76
box breathing, 72, 173
brain physiology, 23
breast cancer prevention, 42
breathing, 71–72, 74, 173
broccoli, 144
burst training, 163
By the Numbers approach, 114–15,
   119–25

C

caffeine, 54–55, 73, 89, 139, 169
calories, 80–81, 111, 120–23
Campos, Marcelo, 44–45

carbohydrates, 13–15, 37, 78, 111,
   112, 119–20
caution foods, 112–13, 118, 125
CBD (cannabidiol) oil, 172
cellular-repair processes, 41
chicken, 135
Chinese restaurant cuisines, 151
Chipotle, 152
Christ-confidence, 180–81
cinnamon, 68
Classic Christianity (George), 23
cleansing drink, 126
cleansing symptoms, 72–74, 83
coaching, virtual, 127
coconut milk, 55
coconut oil, 138, 143
coffee, 54–55, 138–39
Cole, Will, 36
collagen, 75, 143
condiments, 63–64
corn, 98–99
corn test, 75–76
cranberries, 144
cranberry drink, 69, 84, 127
cross-training exercise, 162
Crum, Alia, 21–22
cucumbers, 144
cured meats, 136

D

daily checklist, Elimination Phase,
   79
daily practice, self-talk, 31–33
daily worksheet
   Discovery Phase, 104–5
   Keep It Simple, 116–19
   By the Numbers, 123–25

Recipe and Ingredient Index

More About Danna

At age sixty-six, Danna still describes herself as a "work in progress." She has a diverse professional background as a registered nurse specializing in labor and delivery, a corporate marketing manager for a Fortune 100 company, a fitness professional, a lifestyle coach, and a talk-radio host, to name a few of her roles.

She is also a popular retreat and conference speaker and the author of several books, including *Change Your Habits, Change Your Life* and *What Happened to My Life?* Of all her roles, she considers those of wife, mom, and grandmother to be the most important.

Danna and her husband, Lew, have four adult children and four grandchildren and live in Alpine, California. In their latest life adventure, they moved to a more rural area, where they are taking on new hobbies. From hiking and working in her garden to tending to her thirteen chickens and taking her dogs on long walks, Danna is living the active, "ageless" lifestyle that keeps her young in body, soul, and spirit!

More About Robyn

A lifelong entrepreneur, Robyn was drawn to health and nutrition in her early twenties and has been passionate about helping people achieve wellness for the past three decades. She is an advanced clinical weight-loss practitioner and has worked with cutting-edge nutritional companies, receiving training from some of the top doctors and scientists in the industry. She has taken her knowledge and passed it along to thousands through seminars, workshops, and one-on-one coaching.

At age fifty-two, her thirst to discover the most accurate and innovative health information is unquenchable. Her comprehensive research greatly enhances the podcasts, videos, and programs that she creates with Danna to equip and encourage women, especially those in the "ageless" category!

Robyn lives with her husband, Rob, in San Diego. A huge animal lover, she likes to spend lots of time on the canyon trails of California riding her horse, Bailey.

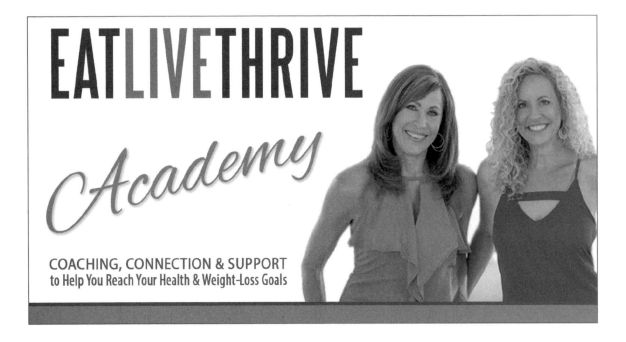

EATLIVETHRIVE *Academy*

COACHING, CONNECTION & SUPPORT
to Help You Reach Your Health & Weight-Loss Goals

STUDIES PROVE THAT LASTING WEIGHT LOSS IS BEST ACHIEVED WHEN A WOMAN HAS:

- A strong support system and accountability
- A strategy for changing her habits through changing her mind-set
- A lifestyle eating plan that is both sustainable and enjoyable

The Eat Live Thrive Academy helps women do just that! It is an added level of support for our *Eat, Live, Thrive Diet* readers who desire direct coaching and accountability from Danna and Robyn. You will have direct access to your coaches and the opportunity to fine-tune your lifestyle plan to meet your unique needs. For a very low monthly or annual membership fee, you will receive the kind of personalized attention that could cost hundreds from a face-to-face nutritionist, exercise trainer, or life coach.

WHAT MAKES OUR MEMBERSHIP PROGRAM UNIQUE?

- Live weekly coaching sessions with Danna and Robyn via video or phone (recorded)
- Daily connection for questions and encouragement via private Facebook Support Group
- Personalized approach to customize your diet and lifestyle
- Interaction with successful members for encouragement and support
- Comprehensive coaching to help you change your habits from the inside out
- Access to the private Academy website with video modules and resources
- Highly affordable membership

"Our Eat Live Thrive coaches, Danna and Robyn, rock! A very personal experience for all of our life struggles: weight, health, beauty advice, etc.! It feels like we're just a bunch of girlfriends going through all of this together!"
—TRACEY RENAUD

"The Eat Live Thrive Academy gives me the coaching and encouragement I need to be my healthiest self and the accountability to stick with my good choices."
—DIANA METZ

"The Academy truly makes me feel like I can achieve my goals with ongoing support even when I sometimes feel like quitting. They always encourage me to just keep going."
—EMMA KELLN

"The Eat Live Thrive Academy has provided me with the tools, resources, accountability, and support I need to make healthy changes in my life."
—TRACEY REYNOLDS

"I've lost over 24 pounds with the Eat, Live, Thrive Diet. For me, the Academy is my one-stop shop with a wide variety of support ranging from diet and exercise to supplements, skincare, and even some fashion advice on occasion!"
—SANDI FEENEY

"The Academy has brought me out of my isolation and from feeling like no one cares. Danna and Robyn do care and provide excellent resources, support, encouragement, and accountability for me to be the best me I can be through healthy lifestyle choices."
—SHELLEY ARNSTAD

For more info or to enroll, visit EatLiveThriveAcademy.com